SUCCESSFUL MOVEMENT CHALLENGES

MOVEMENT ACTIVITIES FOR THE DEVELOPING CHILD

by

JACK CAPON

SECOND EDITION

EDITOR
Frank Alexander

EDITORIAL ASSISTANT
Diane Alexander

ARTIST
John Lewis

Published by FRONT ROW EXPERIENCE, 540 Discovery Bay Blvd., Byron, Calif. 94514

4,137 BOOKS IN PRINT AS OF 1993

ISBN 0-915256-07-X

Published

by

FRONT ROW EXPERIENCE
540 Discovery Bay Blvd.
Byron, California 94514

CONTENTS

IN DEDICATION

This book is dedicated to the hundreds of elementary school and pre-school classroom teachers with whom I have had the pleasure of working since 1958. I have found these teachers to be receptive to new ideas and more than willing to meet the challenge of teaching physical education, if given needed support and tools to work with.

In some States and school districts, trained physical education teachers are employed to teach elementary school physical education, but this is the exception rather than the rule. The elementary and pre-school classroom teacher is generally expected to be "all things to all children", and all too often has not received any training in teaching movement education activities. It is hoped that this book will serve as a valuable resource for assisting teachers in meeting the physical needs of students in their classes.

ABOUT THE AUTHOR

Jack Capon is known nationally and internationally for his "practical" application of Movement Education to the classroom environment. By means of his numerous workshops conducted throughout the world, Jack Capon has shown how teachers and others interested in Movement Education can start their own successful program. This book is a further effort by Jack to provide teachers and schools with a practical approach to organizing the physical education program in the elementary grades.

Jack Capon has been active in Movement Education since the early 1960's. His present position is with the Alameda City School District of California as Coordinator For Physical Education. The nationally recognized Perceptual-Motor Program he developed in Alameda now serves as a model for similar Programs in operation throughout the U.S., Canada, and Australia.

Jack Capon has been very active in Movement Education, not only in the practical sense of being "out in the field", but through his many other activities. He served 4 years (1968-72) on the Perceptual-Motor Task Force of the American Association for Health, Physical Education, Recreation and Dance. He was elected National Chairman of the Elementary Physical Education Section of AAHPERD in 1972. Jack served as a consultant for the film THINKING-MOVING-LEARNING in 1970, which was his first major effort to promote Movement Education by means of the media in the United States. In 1971, he served as co-producer of the record album PERCEPTUAL-MOTOR RHYTHM GAMES which combined music with perceptual-motor activities. In 1974, he wrote the first edition of his popular book, PERCEPTUAL-MOTOR LESSON PLANS, LEVEL-1, plus several other booklets on specific types of equipment activities. In 1977, he wrote PERCEPTUAL-MOTOR LESSON PLANS, LEVEL-2, which was designed for students that have successfully completed the Level-1 book. Jack's work has been further publicized through numerous articles in various nationally circulated educational magazines. His contribution to both the State of California and the national education scene was recognized in 1978 when the California Association of Health, Physical Education, Recreation, and Dance presented him with their State Honor Award. And the American Association of Health, Physical Education, Recreation, and Dance presented him with the City and County Director's Honor Award. Further recognition was bestowed on Jack Capon in 1982 when the California Association of School Administrators (ACSA, Region 6) selected him as the "Outstanding Administrator" of the year.

INTRODUCTION

Education today is focused on the individual child, the child's estimated potential, progress towards achieving that potential, and the additional skills and knowledge needed to reach that potential. Each kind of activity in the physical education program has something to contribute to this development, but the order of priorities for teaching these different activities has changed considerably. We have ceased to think in terms of skills which we would like to have the child develop for the near future, or for use as an adult. Instead, we are saying, "How can we help now? What does a child need in order to be?"

There is a growing amount of research concerned with the development of the human personality which makes it quite evident that what children think of themselves and how they see themselves as individuals are factors which, to a large extent, control learning. How does a child arrive at feeling adequate or inadequate, successful or unsuccessful, a desirable person or one to be barely tolerated? Self-concept comes from the totality of experiences and how he/she performs in all these situations. In the physical education program, Movement Challenges have a high potential for providing each child with a positive self-image.

What are Movement Challenges? They can take on many different characteristics, but basically they involve learning through moving, moving purposefully in ways which make positive contributions to knowledge of self and the physical environment. Through these experiences, the child develops skills in the use of the body, in the use of objects, and in the manipulation and mastery of space. Along with new skills and knowledge come attitudes which relate to the ability to solve problems, and to work with others to achieve mutually desired goals. Through Movement Challenges, the *whole child*, as well as the *whole class*, can be involved all the time. The learning process becomes a whole one, rather than a fragmented one.

A primary approach to presenting Movement Challenges is that of exploration and problem solving through the presentation of a series of challenges which allow *every child to succeed to some extent*. It is the instructor's responsibility to see that this feeling of accomplishment and success pervades each lesson. The tools are leading questions or invitations to explore movement for which there are many many answers or responses. Phrases such as, "Can you...?", "Show me how...", "Is there another way?", "Try it with a friend!", etc., become the key to motivating children to think and respond with actions which reflect improved skill and movement awareness. In this non-competitive environment, children are normally eager to participate because preconceived standards are not set and total involvement reduces the risks of students becoming self-conscious and critical of each other. As skill is acquired, the degree of difficulty of challenges presented is readily adaptable to the student's interest and ability.

The goal is to motivate children to continue trying to solve problems! The goal is to keep adding to their ability to make judgements and to perform successfully in response to these judgements. The goal is to help children *think and do* and, in the process, *learn*! The teacher or leader is constantly encouraging, praising, noting progress, and watching for evidence of creative thinking.

The evaluation of success is made at once by the children, and as they add one small success to another, one new skill to another, grow in their ability to listen, follow cues, and create; they become what each one of us would have them become: alert, confident, thinking, sharing, creating individuals. It is in this way that Movement challenges become an important dimension in the education of today's children!

USE OF MATERIAL IN THIS BOOK

Children enjoy the fun and excitement of physical activity when they are challenged to perform movement tasks that arouse their curiosity and at the same time assure them of a large number of successful experiences. The hundreds of movement challenges presented in this book have been field tested in elementary schools throughout the United States since 1965. The author has, in addition, successfully introduced these activities to teachers and parents in numerous workshops conducted in several different countries. A diverse selection of movement challenges requiring no equipment are offered, as well as a focus on challenges which utilize a wide variety of equipment items.

Teachers should begin the use of this material by carefully assessing the present motor development level of students and determining individual needs. The Motor Development Evaluation Scale presented in this book, or an appropriate comparable screening instrument, can be used for this purpose. Once the evaluation process is completed, teachers can then select movement challenges from this book which are at the present performance level of participating students.

Activities should be selected with the basic broad goals of a physical education or movement program constantly in focus. These basic goals normally include, but are not limited to:

1) Development and refinement of balance skills
2) Development and refinement of locomotor skills
3) Development and refinement of manipulation skills
4) Development and refinement of body/space awareness skills

Every possible effort should be expended to insure that the overall movement program consists of an integrated curriculum which will assist all children in meeting the stated goals. Movement Challenges are organized within this book for easy referral and selection by the teacher. The intent is to provide practical and easy-to-use resource material which will enable the user to challenge children to move within an environment permeated by fun and excitement as well as success.

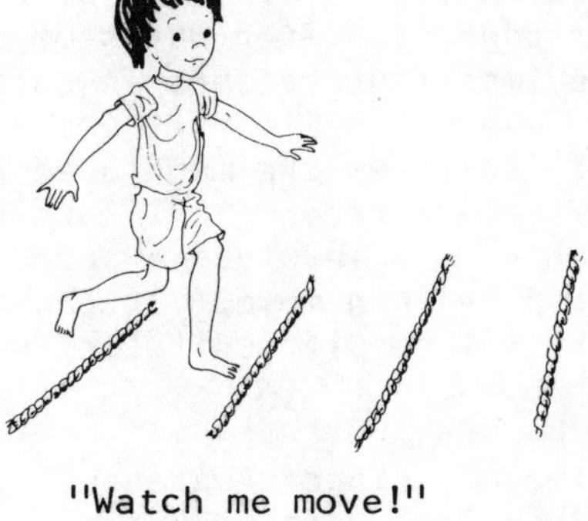

"Watch me move!"

CONCEPTS OF MOTOR DEVELOPMENT

Motor coordination is normally classified under 2 major categories, gross motor and fine motor. Gross Motor coordination refers to acquiring more efficient use of the skeletal or large muscles in producing coordinated and effective total body action. Fine Motor coordination results from the development of the delicate or small muscle systems to the degree that they can perform specific small movements (that is, cutting, grasping, catching, etc.). Gross Motor coordination allows the child to master the environment by transporting the body with control through space, while Fine Motor coordination allows the child to master the environment by efficiently manipulating objects. In this book you will be exposed to a wide variety of movement activities which have been carefully selected to assist children in refining both Gross Motor and Fine Motor coordination skills.

When we examine the process by which children develop their motor coordination, the relationship of perception to physical activity takes on primary importance. The body contains over 600 muscles which enable us to move and communicate. The brain controls the muscles of the body, and the ability of the brain to send the proper signals to these muscles depends on many factors. One of the most important factors is previous experience. Walking, climbing, balancing, catching, and writing are examples of motor activities that depend on the brain's ability to accurately interpret sensory information. Each of these successful physical acts are dependent upon thousands of previous sensorimotor experiences.

One's capacity to receive, interpret, and respond successfully to sensory information is commonly referred to as Perceptual-Motor Ability. Perception is the receiving or input system while motor refers to output or responsive movements. The environment that the child is placed into will determine the type of sensory stimuli that must be processed by the brain. In movement programs, participants receive information primarily through the visual, tactile, kinesthetic, auditory, and vestibular senses. All conscious and controlled movement depends on one's ability to interpret sensory input.

The abilities which enable children to properly respond to sensory information are referred to as Perceptual-Motor Abilities. A Perceptual-Motor Ability could therefore be defined as a capacity for organizing sensory information. These abilities include, but are not limited to, balance, body and space awareness, laterality, directionality, hand-eye and foot-eye coordination, and ocular motor control. Attributes of movement such as agility, strength, flexibility, and rhythm become important factors in successful muscle response.

Some of these Perceptual-Motor Abilities are mentioned on numerous occasions within this publication and, therefore, deserve further clarification. Body Image is the individual's concept of the body and its parts. It involves awareness of the physical structure of the body, and how the body and its parts can move. If the child does not know and understand itself as a physical being, it will be difficult for the child to use its body with comfort and control.

Closely associated with Body Image is Space Awareness. Not only must a child develop an understanding of oneself as a physical person, but must continually face the challenge of moving one's body through ever changing environments. These environments impose space barriers within which the child must feel secure and confident in transporting one's body.

Balance is the ability to assume and maintain any body position against the forces of gravity. It envolves many different sensory modalities, internal organisms, and muscle groups interacting together to control one's body position in space. Balance is challenged through creating imbalance. Children should be presented challenges which place them in positions which require adjustments in the center of gravity to maintain equilibrium. The 3 main classifications of balance which are important in the child's development are: dynamic or moving balance, static or stationary balance, and object balance.

Laterality is internal awareness of the difference between right and left. It centers on the ability to control the 2 sides of the body together, separately, or in opposition to each other. Bilateral movements involve the use of both sides of the body in a simultaneous and parallel fashion as in catching a ball with 2 hands. Unilateral movements involve the use of one side of the body or one limb on that body side as in bouncing a ball with one hand. Cross-Laterality is the simultaneous use of different limbs on opposite sides of the body as in walking where arms and legs move in opposition to each other.

Directionality is a term that often is confused with Laterality. It refers to external awareness of left and right, or the projection of space outside the body. It includes knowledge of directions in relation to right and left, in and out, up and down, etc. It enables the child to properly perceive the position of its body in space in relation to people and objects in the immediate environment.

As the child interacts with the environment through planned movement or natural play experiences, the opportunity to refine these and other perceptual-motor abilities is normally present. Organized movement programs should serve as an extension of the child's natural play environment. Unfortunately, society has managed to rapidly decrease developmental movement opportunities for children. Television, housing and land costs, over protective parents, and our mechanized life styles have all taken their toll on physical activity for children. Obviously this has strong implications for movement programs.

Samuel Gridley Howe wrote, "Do not too much regard bumps on the forehead, rough scratches, or bloody noses; even these have their good influences. At worse, they affect only the bark, and not the system like the rust of inaction."

Planned movement opportunities for children should vary between open-ended problem solving challenges such as, "How many different ways can you move your body?", to those tasks which are highly structured as would be the case in directing a child to toss bean bags into bicycle tires. Using different approaches takes into consideration that children learn in many ways and individual needs are not all the same. The greater the variety of motor experiences children are exposed to, the more opportunities for sensory stimulation and learning.

Motor activities which contribute to the child's exploration of the environment are perhaps the most meaningful. It is through exploration that the child gains initial information about the environment. These motor exploration activities should involve not only movement through space, but also the opportunity for manipulation of objects. In general, Gross Motor patterns permit exploration of space while Fine Motor patterns permit exploration of objects. Movement activities should be carefully selected in terms of the contribution they can make to the total development of the child, and not just for the sake of activity as so often is the case. Motor development is too important to leave to chance!

An anonymous writer once wrote: "I saw tomorrow look at me
Through little children's eyes
And thought how carefully we'd plan
If only we were wise."

Active physical involvement is a must for motor learning to take place. The teacher or leader should plan movement experiences that insure a high degree of involvement on the part of all children. Much too often the movement environment becomes the "spot-light" for the physically gifted while the motor deficient child becomes a passive spectator. Programs which focus on a game approach have a tendency to contribute to such a destructive climate. Good movement programs help each child develop and refine basic motor skills in an environment that is reassuring to the point that new tasks are eagerly engaged in without the fear of failure.

It should be pointed out that equipment plays an important role in helping children to develop basic motor skills. Equipment serves as a catalyst for movement, and helps make the program challenging and exciting. However, there is no magic in equipment. The magic is in the child, and is brought out in the human interaction between teacher or parent, and the child. Children need guidance in the correct use of equipment. They need equipment which is appropriate to their size, strength, and coordination. The more equipment available, the more involvement of children, and hopefully, a greater opportunity for learning.

A time-honored theory states: "Motor development is the foundation of child development." If this is true, then all of us who work with children have an obligation to provide comprehensive motor development programs so that no child will want for such vital experiences. It is also generally accepted that children who are successful with movement challenges develop an "I Can" attitude. This evaluation of self in comparison to what one can do is a primary means of acquiring a positive self-image.

Each child must learn for oneself what the body can do, and how and where the body moves. The learning can only take place by doing! The "doing" should be guided by aware, informed, and knowledgeable teachers and parents. Every child deserves the right to become master of one's physical self. There is no more fundamental right than the "Right To Move" with confidence and joy.

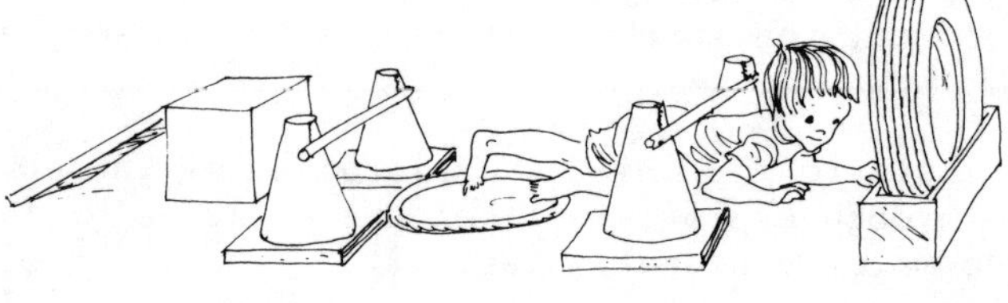

OBSERVATION OF MOVEMENT

Although a motor evaluation scale is included in this book, its use will not be totally effective unless teachers acquire skills in observation of movement behavior. The brief discussion which follows should serve to improve competencies in this important area. Observing the moving child with insight is not an easy assignment. Movement takes place very rapidly and the tendency is to evaluate the total act itself rather than its parts.

One of the first movement characteristics which can be observed is the use of the arms and legs in a coordinated action. Do they work together to accomplish the task in the most efficient manner? For example, in walking and running the arms and legs must work in opposition to each other to secure proper weight distribution. This is a cross-lateral action. This is also true in throwing a ball where the child throwing with the right hand should step forward with the left foot. In jumping, the arms and legs work together in bilateral coordination. The arms initiate the action as they swing forward and up as the legs are extended. This coordinated effort enables proper force to be exerted and organizes total body action. As the knees, ankles, and hips flex to absorb or cushion the landing, the arms swing down to help stabilize body position.

Proper weight transference is another important factor which leads to efficient movement. The teacher must be able to observe whether or not the child demonstrates correct body positioning to maintain control and balance. Examples of common errors would be head and shoulders leaning too far forward, or body leaning strongly to one side. Many children reveal very rigid body action which inhibits the flow of movement and causes poor weight distribution. In throwing and striking activities, the weight must be allowed to shift forward from the back foot onto the forward foot. Proper weight transference is a vital factor in establishing body balance. Balance is the foundation for all successful movement.

In catching balls or other objects the teacher must first look for proper preparation on the part of the receiver. Do the hands form a "pocket" ready to receive the ball? Are the fingers relaxed and spread? The 2nd phase of catching is the actual receiving and controlling of the ball. This involves watching the ball into the hands, and cushioning the ball in towards the body to properly absorb the force of the throw.

Inability to impart the proper amount of force and effort is a deficiency which leads to poor motor performance on the part of many children. This is directly related to kinesthetic awareness or sometimes referred to as "muscle sense". Throwing is a motor act in which poor application of force is a common error. The child throws too hard or in some cases too softly. In locomotor tasks such as in jumping, it is not uncommon to observe the correct coordination of body parts, but poor performance can still result due to an inability to apply adequate force to the act. An example of this can be seen in the challenge of jumping over a low cross bar. The child must be able to apply enough force to propel the body upward and forward to clear the bar. Poor performance could be related to inadequate muscular strength or even faulty integration of visual and kinesthetic information which is a common perceptual-motor deficiency.

Another key assessment factor in movement involves the child's ability to adequately judge space and distance. This becomes of special importance when the child must move in relation to other children and/or objects within a given environment. The teacher should note whether or not the child must give excessive amounts of visual attention to obstacles, as well as efficiency in making quick, accurate changes in body positioning as the child moves through space. We speak of this latter skill in terms of agility. The teacher must be able to observe the child's ability to accurately judge the position of obstacles as the child goes under, over, through, around, between, etc. Also, can the child move without interferring with other children's movements? Can the child move comfortably with a partner, or in a group activity?

A commonly overlooked movement characteristic which the teacher can easily learn to analyze is one of time. In other words, is the child able to make adequate adjustments in the speed of movements to insure quality and control? Many children display awkward movements due to an inability to impart necessary variations in speed such as moving faster or slower. In any given task this could involve a deficiency in processing sensory information. The muscles must be made aware that a change in speed is needed for a successful motor response.

As one assesses an individual's movement behavior it becomes apparent that proper use of space, time, and force along with a well-developed sense of body awareness and balance become the basic characteristics of successful motor actions. These are the common ingredients which, when correctly integrated, enable the child to develop purposeful and controlled movement patterns.

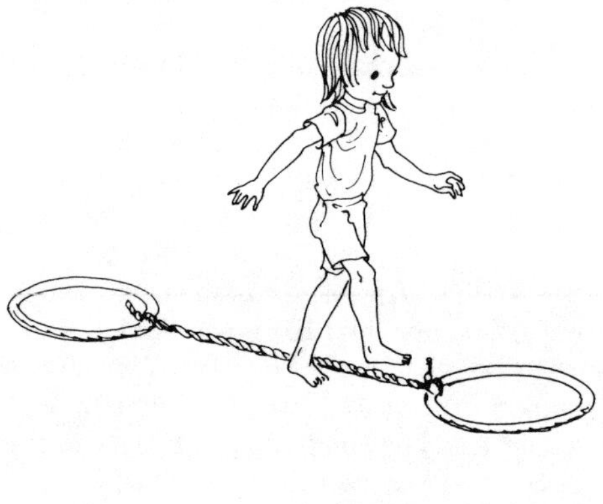

TERMINOLOGY

The following terms are useful in evaluating your students on the Evaluation Scale which follows.

BODY IMAGE
The individual's concept of his or her body and its parts. The concept involves the knowledge of: a) the physical structure of the body and its parts; b) the movements and functions of the body and its parts; and c) the position of the body and its parts in relation to each other and to other objects. It forms a base for acquiring an adequate self-concept.

BALANCE
The ability to assume and maintain any body position against the force of gravity. Maintenance of balance results from the interaction of the muscles working to keep the body on its base.

VISUAL-MOTOR CONTROL
Refers to the ability to successfully integrate visual and motor responses into a physical action. It enables an individual to control movement, and move easily and smoothly from place to place.

COORDINATION
The ability of the body to integrate the action of the muscles of the body to accomplish a specific movement or a series of skilled movements in the most efficient manner.

PROPRIOCEPTION
The awareness of muscular movement and position of the body in space.

GROSS-MOTOR COORDINATION
Results from the development of the skeletal or large muscles to produce efficient total body movement.

FINE-MOTOR COORDINATION
The coordinated use of small muscles resulting from the development of the muscles to the degree that they can perform specific small movements such as cutting, writing, grasping, and so on.

SUSTAINED MOVEMENTS
Motor skills executed consecutively for a number of times or continued for an interval of time.

SPACE AWARENESS (SPATIAL ORIENTATION)
Involves the ability to select a reference point to stabilize functions and to organize objects into correct perspective. It involves knowledge of the body and its position, as well as the positions of other people and objects in relation to one's body in space. Closely associated with body image.

LATERALITY

Internalizing the awareness of: a) the difference between right and left; and b) how far right and how far left various activities are centered. It is the ability to control the 2 sides of the body together or separately and is the motor basis for spatial concepts. Bilateral movements involve the use of both sides of the body in a simultaneous and parallel fashion as in catching a ball with 2 hands. Unilateral movements involve the use of one side of the body or one limb on that body side as in bouncing a ball with one hand. Cross-laterality is the simultaneous use of different limbs on opposite sides of the body as in walking where arms and legs move in opposition to each other.

DIRECTIONALITY

Often confused with laterality. An awareness of space outside of the body and involves: a) knowledge of directions in relation to right and left, in and out, and up and down; b) the projection of one's self in space; and c) the judging of distances between objects.

HAND-EYE COORDINATION

Refers to one's ability to use his or her eyes and hands together to accomplish a task.

FOOT-EYE COORDINATION

Refers to one's ability to use his or her eyes and feet together to accomplish a task.

OCULAR PURSUIT

Ability of the eyes to work together in following (tracking) a moving object or in focusing from one object to another.

KINESTHESIS

One's awareness of muscular movement and expenditure of energy during the performance of a skill.

PERCEPTUAL-MOTOR SKILLS

Those skills which indicate the interrelationships between the perceptual or sensory processes and motor activity and the ability of the individual to receive, interpret, and respond accurately to stimuli, either internal or external. Perceptual-motor learning involves all senses: seeing, hearing, touching, tasting, smelling, and moving or kinesthesis. Also know as "Sensory-Motor Skills".

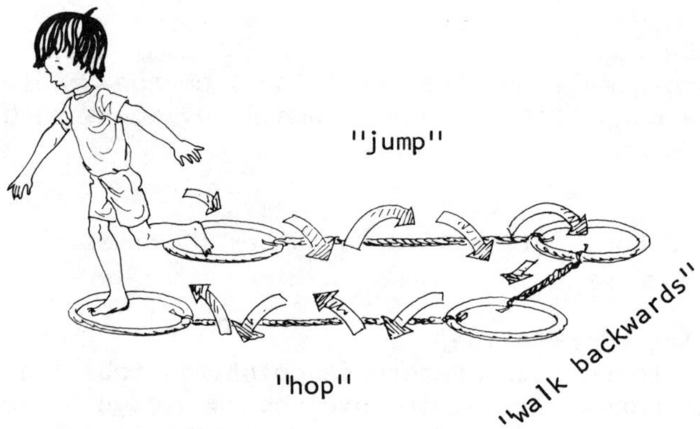

MOTOR DEVELOPMENT EVALUATION SCALE

Before beginning any comprehensive program in motor development, participants should be assessed as to their strengths and weaknesses. Obviously there are countless numbers of screening tasks and surveys which are available for use as an assessment instrument. This "Motor Evaluation Scale" is provided for teachers because it is easy to administer, takes only a limited amount of instruction time, and provides information (as recorded on the "Record Sheet") which teachers can easily use to plan purposeful program activities. It also provides teachers with a tool which may be used to evaluate student progress and program effectiveness.

GENERAL INSTRUCTIONS

1) Tests are designed so that they may be administered as part of the physical education class period.

2) Do not tell the students they are being "tested". Make the screening a natural part of your physical education period.

3) Students are given an "S" for *Satisfactory Performance*, and an "N" for *Needs Improvement*.

4) Students receiving an "N" should be retested in the middle and/or at the end of your Movement Program.

5) Demonstration of test items to show correct response is permissible. You are observing performance, not testing ability to interpret verbal directions.

6) If judgement of a student's performance is uncertain, you may wish to have the student repeat the activity.

7) Test items may be administered over a period of a few weeks, or over a period of a few days at the teacher's discretion.

8) Remember...the main purpose of the screening program is to "look" at each student as an individual, and as a result, plan program activities which will take into account individual needs.

TASK (1) BODY PARTS

PERFORMANCE OBJECTIVES

By touching specific body parts, student demonstrates body image.

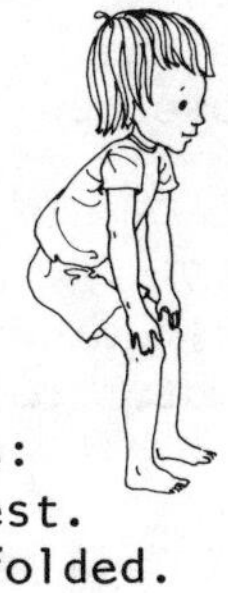

(knees)

CHALLENGES

Ask a student (or students) to stand facing you at a distance of about 10 feet. The student is asked to touch the following body parts: knees, shoulders, hips, head, feet, eyes, elbows, mouth, neck, and chest. If students are tested in a group, their eyes must be closed or blindfolded.

EVALUATION

If a student makes more than one error in identification, is slow or has to "feel" around to find parts, mark an "N" for *Needs Improvement*.

TASK (2) WALKING BOARD

PERFORMANCE OBJECTIVES

By walking forward on a low walking board with eyes focused on the teacher's hand held at eye level, student demonstrates balance, laterality and visual-motor control.

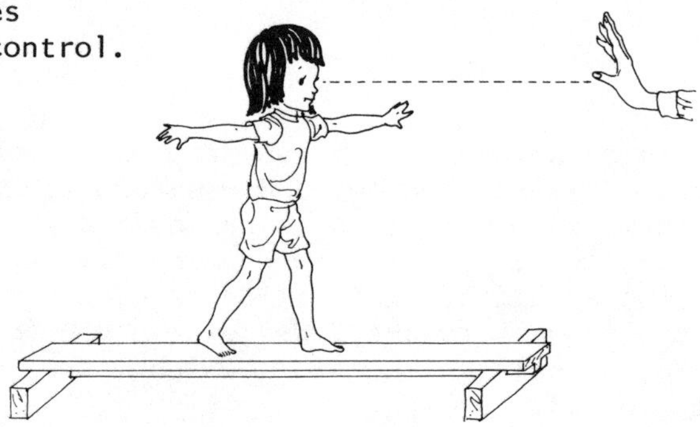

EQUIPMENT

Low walking board.

CHALLENGES

1) Walk slowly forward on the board towards me.
2) Keep your eyes focused on my hand as you walk forward.

EVALUATION

If a student shows any difficulty such as stepping off board, sliding feet, pausing frequently, or uses a fast walk to avoid losing balance, mark an "N" for *Needs Improvement*.

TASK (3) HOPPING

PERFORMANCE OBJECTIVES

By pausing, and hopping on first the right foot then the left, student demonstrates gross-motor coordination, balance and ability to sustain movement.

EQUIPMENT

None.

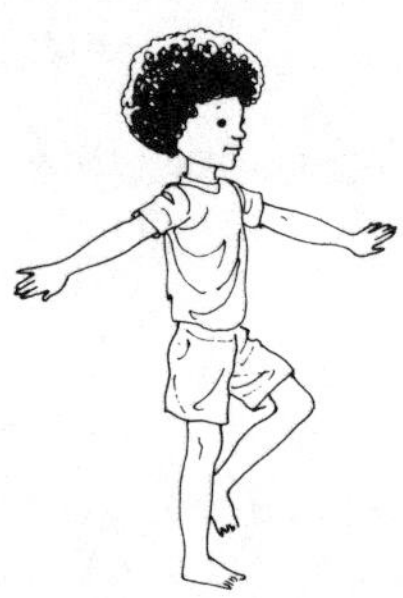

CHALLENGES

1) Stand on your *right* foot for 5 seconds facing away from me.
2) Hop forward 5 times without stopping.
3) Turn and stand facing me with both feet on the floor.
4) Stand on your *left* foot for 5 seconds.
5) Hop forward towards me 5 times without stopping.

EVALUATION

If opposite foot touches ground while either stationary or hopping, or postural shift is not smooth, lacks rhythm, loses control, etc., mark an "N" for *Needs Improvement*.

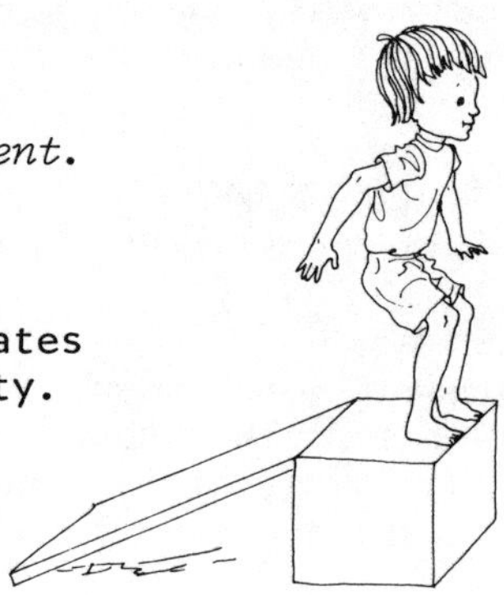

TASK (4) JUMP AND LAND

PERFORMANCE OBJECTIVES

By jumping and landing from a jump box, student demonstrates gross-motor coordination, dynamic balance and bilaterality.

EQUIPMENT

Jump box and mats.

CHALLENGES

1) Take jumping position on jump box with your feet about shoulder distance apart.
2) Jump off the box with both of your feet leaving it at the same time.

3) Land with both of your feet touching down at the same time without losing your balance.

EVALUATION

If both feet do not leave jump box at the same time and land at the same time, or if student is unable to hold balance upon landing, mark an "N" for *Needs Improvement.*

TASK (5) OBSTACLE COURSE

PERFORMANCE OBJECTIVES

By going over, under and between obstacles, student demonstrates spatial orientation and body awareness.

EQUIPMENT

6 chairs and 2 yardsticks.

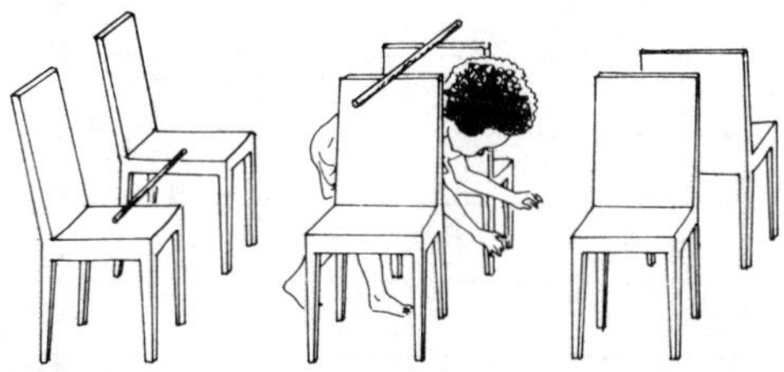

CHALLENGES

Chairs can be substituted for cross bars as shown. However, cross bars which can be adjusted are best. Low cross bar should be at knee height. High cross bar should be at shoulder height.

1) Step over the low cross bar without touching it.
2) Walk under the high cross bar without touching it.
3) Walk between the 2 chairs without touching them. (Place 2 chairs back to back and close enough so that the student must turn sideways to get through without touching.)

EVALUATION

If student over-estimates or under-estimates space by more than a few inches, or if body contact is made with obstacles, mark an "N" for *Needs Improvement.*

TASK (6) BALL CATCH

PERFORMANCE OBJECTIVES

By attempting to catch a ball thrown in an underhand toss by the teacher, student demonstrates eye-hand coordination and ocular pursuit.

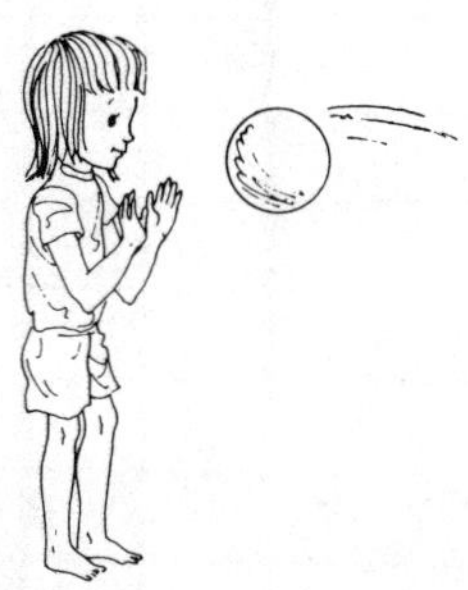

EQUIPMENT

Ball 7 to 8 inches in diameter or equivalent.

CHALLENGES

1) Stand about 10 feet away and face me.
2) Form a catching pocket with your hands.
3) Try to catch the ball I throw to you. You will have 3 chances to catch it.

EVALUATION

If a score of less than 2 catches is made in the 3 trials, mark an "N" for *Needs Improvement.* For a fair catch, ball must be caught with fingers and hands and not with arms and body.

TASK (7) OPTIONAL TESTS

The teacher may wish to run an additional screening check on students. Some examples of optional tests are: Chalkboard, Angels-In-The-Snow, and Creeping.

RECORD TEST RESULTS ON *RECORD SHEET* ON THE FOLLOWING PAGE

MOTOR EVALUATION SCALE

– RECORD SHEET –

MARKING *N = Needs Improvement* *S = Satisfactory*	Task 1 Identify Body Parts		Task 2 Walking Board		Task 3 Hopping		Task 4 Jump & Land		Task 5 Obstacle Course		Task 6 Ball Catch		Task 7 Optional	
NAME	Fall	Spr.	Fall	Spr.	Fall	Spr.	Fall	Spr.	Fall	Spr.	Fall	Spr.	Fall	Spr.
1														
2														
3														
4														
5														
6														
7														
8														
9														
10														
11														
12														
13														
14														
15														
16														
17														
18														
19														
20														
21														
22														
23														
24														
25														
26														
27														
28														
29														
30														

copy this page to make your own record sheet

BODY IMAGE CHALLENGES

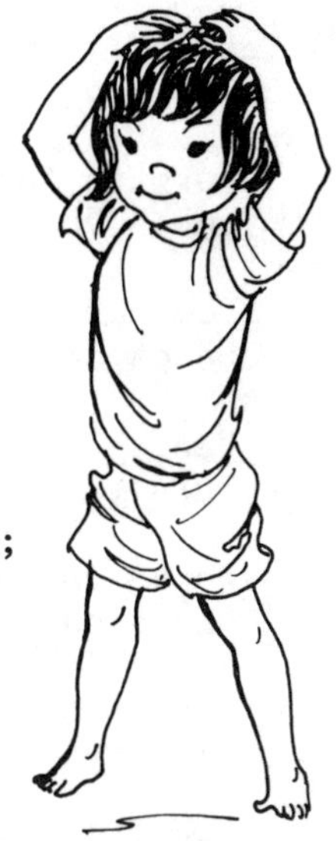

PERFORMANCE OBJECTIVES

By performing the following challenges, student demonstrates body image which includes knowledge of the physical structure of the body and its parts; the movements and functions of the body and its parts; and the position of the body and its parts in relation to each other and to other objects.

EQUIPMENT

None.

GENERAL INFORMATION

Body Image is important in the development of the child's self-concept as well as in coordination. Children need to know themselves as a physical person, and this awareness of the physical body needs to be developed to the highest degree. If a child develops a good image of his or her body, he or she will have a sound base upon which to build the perceptual skills which will be needed in future classroom learning experiences.

CHALLENGES

1) Teacher touches the different body parts starting with the head and says, "This is my head; touch your head." Student then touches head and says, "I am touching my head."
2) Teacher instructs students to place hands on body parts on command. Examples: "Place both hands on your head," "Place both hands on your shoulders," etc.
3) Teacher asks students to close their eyes and then to touch body parts on command. Examples: "Touch your elbows," "Touch your hips," etc.
4) Students are asked to touch body parts using other body parts. Examples below:

chin to chest	wrist to ear	foot to leg
nose to knee	elbow to leg	toes to heel
ear to shoulder	wrist to ankle	head to knee
hands to hips	thumbs to toes	wrist to neck
elbows to knees	fingers to back	arm to leg

5) Students are asked to touch body parts to their surroundings. Examples below:

head to floor	nose to window	fingers to book
hands to wall	knees to chair	elbows to chalkboard
wrists to table	back to floor	toes to wall

6) Teacher instructs the students to move specific body parts on command. Examples below:

Nod your head.	Open and close your eyes.	Shrug your shoulders.
Twist your neck.	Clap your hands.	Snap your fingers.
Bend your elbows.	Wiggle your nose.	Bend your knees.
Rotate your wrists.	Open your mouth.	Stamp your feet.

7) Students are asked to lie on their backs (change body orientation to space) and move various body parts. Examples: "Lift your head," "Lift your legs," "Lift your right hand," "Touch your elbows together," "Touch your left heel to your right knee," etc.

8) Teacher instructs students to touch body parts with their hands in rhythmic sequence as spoken below:

Turn to the right, now if you please,
touch your elbows, and then your knees.

Touch both heels, now your nose.
Hands on your hips, now find your toes.

Hands on shoulders, I ask you please.
Turn to the left, and slap your knees.

Hands on head, also on hair.
Hands on hips, now in the air.

Touch your face, now your feet.
Clap your hands and take your seat.

9) Teacher instructs students to touch body parts with their hands in rhythmic sequence as spoken below:

Hands on your hips, hands on your knees.
Put them behind you, if you please.

Touch your shoulders, touch your nose.
Touch your ears, now touch your toes.

Reach your hands up so high,
make your fingers quickly fly.

While you watch them with your eyes,
on your tip-toes climb to the sky.

Jump forward and backward, if you can.
Find someone near and shake his (her) hand.

10) Teacher instructs students to have fingers on one hand extended. Then with the other hand, students tuck in each finger as named in the rhythmic sequence spoken below:

My fingers are so sleepy.
It's time they went to bed.
So first, you, baby finger,
tuck in your little head.

Ringman, now it's your turn,
and then comes tall man great.
Now pointing finger, hurry,
because it's getting late.

Let's see if all are snuggled in.
No, here's one more to come.
So come, lie close, little brothers,
make room for master thumb.

LOCOMOTOR CHALLENGES

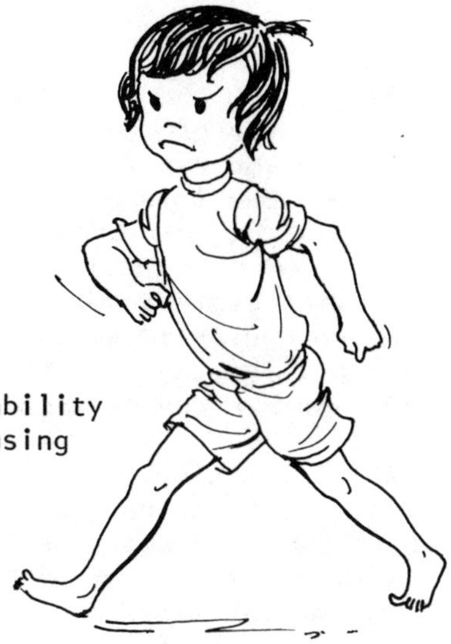

PERFORMANCE OBJECTIVES

By performing the following challenges, student demonstrates ability to move the body through space with control and coordination using a variety of locomotor skills.

EQUIPMENT

None.

GENERAL INFORMATION

There are numerous approaches to providing children with movement experiences. Movement exploration is one method which has proven to be a practical and successful approach for kindergarten and primary grade teachers. The children are presented with a variety of movement challenges which they must react to according to their own interpretation and feelings. Make sure adequate space is provided for freedom and safety of movement. Below you will find outlined basic locomotor (transport) skill areas, and a list of problem solving questions which will lead to purposeful movement experiences.

WALKING CHALLENGES

Stress: Walk tall, shoulders relaxed, feet pointing forward. Look for large spaces to move into!

1) Let's see if you can all walk tall among your classmates with shoulders relaxed and toes pointed forward. (Use a large area.)
2) Avoid all personal contact while walking among classmates within a circle. (Use a smaller area.)
3) Can you walk on your tip toes? How can you keep better balance? (Student raises arms slightly.)
4) Take as few steps as possible to move from one place to another.
5) Who can walk quickly and quietly? (Student moves from one spot to another.)
6) While walking, change direction on a signal, but do not touch anyone.
7) Change direction and show me how you can walk backwards.
8) Can you walk proudly?
9) How can you vary the speed of your walking?
10) On signal, change levels (height) while walking.
11) Change level and direction while walking.
12) Keep hands low while walking at a high level.
13) Keep the hands high while walking at a low level.
14) Can you do a toe-heel walk and maintain your balance?
15) Express your mood while walking. Is it happy, tired, frightened, angry?
16) How would the wind affect the way a person walks?

RUNNING CHALLENGES

Sress: Run on toes and balls of feet with weight slightly forward and feet pointing straight ahead. Be alert!

1) How would you run in place?
2) Who can run to the wall and back? Show me. (If outside, use fence and back, etc.)

3) Can you run high and stay on your toes?
4) Can you use your arms and elbows when you run?
5) Can you run fast, and stop (freeze) on a signal?
6) Who can lift their knees when they run?
7) Can you point your toes when you run?
8) Show me how you can lean forward when you run.
9) What can you do to be in a hurry in the air?
10) How quietly can you run?
11) How low can you run? Can you change from low to high as you run?
12) Who can change speed and direction while they run?

LEAPING CHALLENGES

Stress: Giant run in space followed by an equal leap with both feet and land lightly on foot opposite the take-off foot.

1) Let's take some high running steps.
2) Now let's take some with a leap at the end (a giant run).
3) Let's try for a higher leap and see how lightly we can land.
4) Turn around and run in the opposite direction and see how far you can leap.
5) Who can make the lowest leap?
6) Can you leap with your opposite arm and leg forward as if you were leaping over a log?
7) Who can leap for something high, reaching with both hands?
8) Show me how you can clap your hands over your head as you take a giant leap.
9) Can you leap from side to side in place? (Student goes back and forth over a line or rope.)
10) Who can run and then leap on my signal?

JUMPING CHALLENGES

Stress: Take off on one or 2 feet, but both feet must land at the same time. Use arms in a forward and upward direction.

1) Can you bend your knees and go down?
2) Can you come back up and reach high, higher, higher, etc., ?
3) Can your feet leave the floor? Show me! Good, now you are jumping!
4) Can you jump high, higher, higher?
5) Can you jump high, but land very low?
6) Can you jump forwards?
7) Show me how lightly you can land on your feet as you jump forward.
8) Who can jump backwards?
9) Show me how you would jump forward and then backward.
10) How would you jump sideways? Can you jump from side to side?
11) Who can jump forward, backward, and then sideways?
12) How would you make 5 small jumps each time landing lightly on your toes?
13) Show me how far forward you can jump. This is called a long jump!
14) Can you long jump and throw your arms forward and upward as you jump?

HOPPING CHALLENGES

Stress: Take off, and land on one foot. Use same foot for take-off and landing.

1) Who can jump up and down on 2 feet?
2) Show me if you can take off and land on the same foot. This is called a hop.
3) Now let's try the other foot.
4) Let's hop forward around a circle formation, and change to your other foot every 5 hops.
5) Show me how high you can hop for a few times.
6) How low can you be and still hop?
7) Let's see what great big hops you can make.
8) How lightly can you hop?
9) Try leaning forward slightly as you hop.

10) Who can use their arms to help lift their body as they hop?
11) Who can hop backwards?
12) Show me who can hop sideways.
13) Can you return on the other foot?
14) Try folding your arms while you hop.
15) Can you clasp your arms behind you while you hop?
16) Who can hop with your arms extended out in front of your body?
17) Can you hop along in a zigzag line?
18) Until I stop you, try jumping 3 times, then hopping 3 times (continue the same pattern).

SKIPPING CHALLENGES

Stress: Step-hop rhythm with a changing of the lead foot; not too fast.

1) Can you hop lightly on one foot and then the other without moving forward?
2) Can you hop lightly on one foot, then the other, and move slowly around in a circle?
3) Can you hop lightly on one foot, then the other, and move faster around in a circle? You are now skipping!
4) Can you skip among classmates, changing directions in order to avoid a collision?
5) Can you make your arms move forward and backward while skipping?
6) Let's see you skip backwards. Don't give up, this is a hard challenge!
7) Who can skip in a square? Now try a bigger square!
8) Can you skip in your own little circle? A bigger circle? How about a giant circle?
9) Who can skip low to the ground? Now, how tall can you be while skipping?
10) Let's see you skip, and change your levels: high to low, tall to small, etc.

GALLOP CHALLENGES

Stress: Keep one foot ahead of the other. Push off with the rear foot.

1) Who can walk slowly around in a circle? Show me.
2) Now, can you put one foot in front and pull the other up behind it?
3) Can you change feet and put the other one in front?
4) Who can go a little faster being sure to keep the same foot in front?
5) Show me how fast you can go, but watch your spacing.
6) Can you change the foot that is in front and go faster?
7) Can you try bending your knees a little more and land on the balls of your feet?
8) Now, who can do the same thing and go in the other direction?
9) I wonder who can gallop like a pony. Let's go forward first and then backwards. Try it fast and smoothly. Now gallop! Stop!
10) Can you gallop with a partner?

SLIDING CHALLENGES

Stress: Move to the side; *bend knees*; do *not* cross the feet. It's like a sideward gallop.

1) Let's stand with our feet apart.
2) Show me a way to bring your feet together. Another.
3) Can you hold one foot completely still and slide the other foot to it? Do it several times.
4) Try sliding the other foot over to the foot that is still.
5) Can you move across the floor doing this? You are now sliding!
6) Try going in the opposite direction.
7) Show me how you bend your knees to help you move more quickly?
8) Let's all practice this, moving in different directions.
9) Is sliding an up and down movement or a sideways movement? How can you show this with your arms?
10) Let's all move around the circle this way.
11) Try going in the opposite direction.
12) Can you slide slowly?

13) Can you slide quickly?
14) Try changing your speed from slow to quick as you slide.
15) Show me how you can slide in a smaller circle with good body control.
16) Now, as you move in one direction, we are facing one wall. Can you move in the same direction and on a signal face the opposite wall? Let's all move facing one wall. Now change. Change again.
17) Try taking 4 sliding steps facing one wall and then 4 steps more facing the other wall.
18) Move all the way around the room this way once. Let's do it again.

GENERAL LOCOMOTION CHALLENGES

Stress: Look and think before moving. Student must learn to control movement within a given space.

1) Notice where you are standing.
2) Move away from the home spot; then return when the signal "home" (or whistle) is given.
3) Move farther away from "home" and look in another direction. Return on signal (whistle).
4) Look around to avoid collisions. Run about the area, returning "home" on a signal.
5) Look at a spot away from home. Go to that spot as quickly as possible; then return home.
6) This time find 2 spots away from home. Visit one spot and then the other, returning home as quickly as possible.
7) Move in this (use arm signal) direction in the fastest method you can.
8) Return home quickly.
9) In a low position, move from that direction (use arm signal) until the whistle blows. Come back home in another low position.
10) Find a way to get from here to there (use a gesture), moving from high to low, low to high many times.
11) What can you do that will cause one side to lead as you move from here to there (use gesture)?
12) Come back with the other side leading.
13) Find a place where you have a great amount of room to yourself. Move about that space in the pattern of a large "O".
14) Move in a pattern that will form this (use flash card) shape. (Show a square.)
15) Can you move backward in that same pattern?
16) Is it possible to face in one direction only while moving in the square pattern?
17) Now try to move in the pattern of this shape (show card of triangle).
18) Who can move in the pattern of the letter "C"?
19) Show me the letter "Z".
20) How could you move in the pattern of "X" touching the ground only where you would want to place a line?
21) Make an "X" with your body while standing where you are.
22) Make a pattern of the first letter in your first name.
23) Try moving backward while making the pattern of the first letter in your last name.
24) How would your full first name look if you moved in a pattern to form all the letters?
25) Can you walk in the pattern of the word "walk"?
26) Run in the pattern of the word "run".
27) Stand anywhere on the 4 lines of a square or rectangle. (Use a basketball court or multi-purpose game court, etc.) On signal, walk to the opposite side without touching anyone, in a straight line. You will have to slow down and let another pass at times. Try it while walking faster. Running, skipping, hopping, and sliding.

PARTNER CHALLENGES

Stress: Controlled movements with careful visual guidance.

1) Can you walk far away from your partner without touching anyone? Show me. Now, can you walk back?
2) How will you creep away from your partner and turn and come back to your partner?
3) Can you take long steps away from your partner and make them high when you come back?

4) How can you run away from your partner and find your partner again with one of you high and one low?

Show me how you can change partners quickly.

5) Can you jump away from your partner and jump backwards to your partner?
6) How would you slide away from your partner and slide back to your partner? Show me.
7) Who can gallop away from their partner and then when you get back "freeze" with one hand touching the ground and raise one leg in the air? Show me.
8) Can you skip backward from your partner and then forward to your partner? Show me.
9) Show me how you can join hands with your partner and gallop forward. Now change direction!
10) As a final challenge, discover how many different ways you can balance in place with your partner. Try using different body parts as well as different body positions.

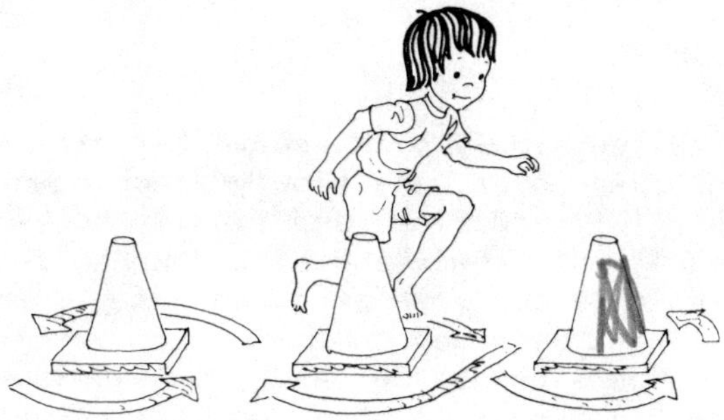

CREATIVE MOVEMENT CHALLENGES

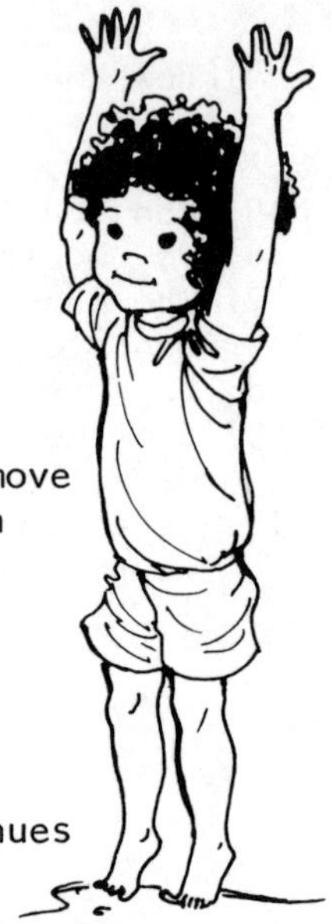

PERFORMANCE OBJECTIVES

By performing the following challenges, student demonstrates ability to move his/her body in imaginative and creative ways. The child becomes more in tune with how the body is capable of moving.

EQUIPMENT

None.

GENERAL INFORMATION

Movement is basic to life. It begins before the child is born and continues through developmental stages into the school environment. Movement to young children means freedom to explore the fascinating world about them. Children need opportunities to explore and discover, and thus to grow creatively. By exploring and probing, a child develops a basic impression of how the body moves. By refining these motions the child discovers how to vary movements or how to control the body. A child who has control over its movements and a good body image is one who will grow in self-confidence.

A variety of purposeful movement experiences are outlined here for the preschool and primary grade teacher.

WARM-UP CHALLENGES

1) Breath in as arms are raised slowly over head. Let air out as arms flop down at sides.
2) Stretch up high on toes, bend over, and slowly reach down and touch toes.
3) Flop arms at sides, then let head flop, and finally body flops forward.
4) Take a big breath. Let it out slowly and sink down to the floor.
5) Stretch up high! How quickly can you let go and drop down to the floor without making a sound? Be soft like a bean bag.
6) Stand still! Stretch up as high as you can. How slowly and softly can you let yourself sink into the floor? Take as long as you want but you must keep moving. Freeze when you reach the floor.

MOVEMENT CHALLENGES

1) How small can you make yourself?
2) How big can you make yourself?
3) Who can make themselves wide?
4) Show me how thin or narrow you can make yourself.
5) Can you make yourself round (like a circle)?
6) How short can you make yourself?
7) Now, can you slowly become a tall building (skyscraper)? Is there a way you can become even taller?
8) Who can place themselves in a position between being small and tall?
9) Can you bounce like a rubber ball?
10) Show me how a top spins.
11) Who can let their body stretch out like a piece of gum?
12) Show me how an elephant's trunk would look when it is swinging.
13) Let's pretend you are the strongest person in the world. Show me how you would push 2 pianos apart.

14) How would a snake look and sound moving through the bushes?
15) Can you twist your body like a pretzel?
16) Who can shake themselves out like a dust mop (or like jelly)?
17) Pretend you are a tree caught in a wind storm. Show me how you would move.
18) How would you look pulling a heavy wagon up a hill?
19) Who can blow themselves up slowly like a balloon, and then let the air out?
20) How would you look walking barefoot over sharp stones and pebbles.
21) Can you tie yourself up into a knot? Can you pull the knot tighter?
22) How does a rocket ship take off? Let's all do it together now, ready, 5, 4, 3, 2, 1, "Blast off!"

NUMBER AND LETTER CHALLENGES

1) Can you make the number "2" using your body?
2) Repeat #1 above by using other numbers such as 1, 3, 4, 6, etc.
3) Let's see who can form the letter capital "C" with their body?
4) Repeat #3 using such capital letters as A, Y, P, L, V, etc.
5) Have the students work with partners and form numbers such as 12, 17, 24, etc.
6) Have students work in small groups and spell out simple words with their bodies such as cat, dog, boy, etc.

BODY AWARENESS CHALLENGES

Work with a rhythm drum and tap out a 4 count beat. Many combinations of 4 body parts can be used in the rhythmic pattern. The student touches the body part and says it aloud or the student moves the body part in rhythm as he or she says it aloud. The 4 count rhythm is constantly maintained. The following sequences are examples to use.

1) Head - Shoulders - Knees - Toes
2) Ears - Nose - Chin - Elbows
3) Hips - Ankles - Feet - Toes
4) Head - Shoulders - Elbows - Wrists
5) Chest - Ribs - Torso - Hips

BUILDING BRIDGE CHALLENGES

Stress: A wide base of support for proper balance.

1) Show me how you make a bridge using your hands and feet to support your body.
2) Now can you make a bridge with your arms and feet?
3) How can you make a bridge using just your legs? Now one leg.
4) Can you make a bridge *over* your head?
5) Show me how to make a bridge *under* your chin?
6) How *high* can you make a bridge?
7) How *low* can you make a bridge?
8) Who can make the bridge another way?
9) Show me how to make a bridge using one arm and one leg.
10) How can you be a Draw Bridge? (You may have to ask what is a Draw Bridge first.)
11) Show me a swinging bridge.
12) Can you make a long bridge?
13) Now show me a short bridge. Can you make it smaller?
14) Who can make any kind of a bridge and hold it while I count to 5?
15) Can you build a bridge over a partner? Now let your partner build the bridge.
16) With your partner, construct different types of bridges. Both of you must form one bridge.

OTHER CHALLENGES

1) *Melting Snowman* - Students demonstrate what happens to a snowman after the sun hits it. Each part of the body starting with the head melts down until the snowman no longer exists. Students can then make a new snowman starting with the toes.

2) *Mirror Images* - Students work with a partner, and one student performs movement patterns slowly while the other student attempts to mirror (imitate) the action. Start with stationary movement, and then have them move into dynamic movement (jumping, turning, swaying, etc.). Add music to provide additional interest and challenge.
3) *Group Movements* - Each group of 7 or 8 students is assigned a particular rhythm pattern on the drum to move to, and also someone or something to imitate. (Example: a giant, elephants, high stepping soldiers, etc.) Whenever a group hears their rhythm pattern they stand and move accordingly. Other groups are kneeling or sitting in an alert position ready to move. The group moving must freeze as soon as a new rhythm pattern is sounded.
4) *Be An Object* - Let each student choose an object: ball, pencil, rope, book, etc. Tell the students to look at their object, feel it, and listen to it. (Does it make a sound?) Using only their bodies, the students must explain what the object is. What can it do, how big is it, how does it move, etc.?
5) *Shadow Pictures* - Students must be able to see their shadows. They must make the hands, head, feet, and other parts of the shadow do different things. They must be able to identify each part of their shadows as the shadows move.
6) *Balloons* - Explain to the students that they are each a big balloon with feet, legs, body, arms, hands, and head. The teacher further explains that the students will be blown up by the teacher. For example: "How does the air come into your body, legs, arms, etc. Show me as I blow you up. Now I will let the air out slowly. This time I am going to prick you with a pin, etc."
7) *Isolations* - Use a record such as the music to "Frenchy Brown" by the Tijuana Brass, etc. Students move one part of their bodies at a time in rhythm with the music. Teacher calls out body parts to be moved. Fingers, shoulders, elbows, knees, hips, etc.
8) *Animal Movements* - Children are challenged to move like different animals such as 4-legged, 3-legged, one-legged, etc. Interest is added when they must create the sound of their animals as the children move. Music can be added for increased motivation and sensory involvement. Use challenges such as, "Can you move like an animal whose name begins with the letter 'C'?", or "With a partner can you create an animal that no one has ever seen before? What sound would it make?, etc."

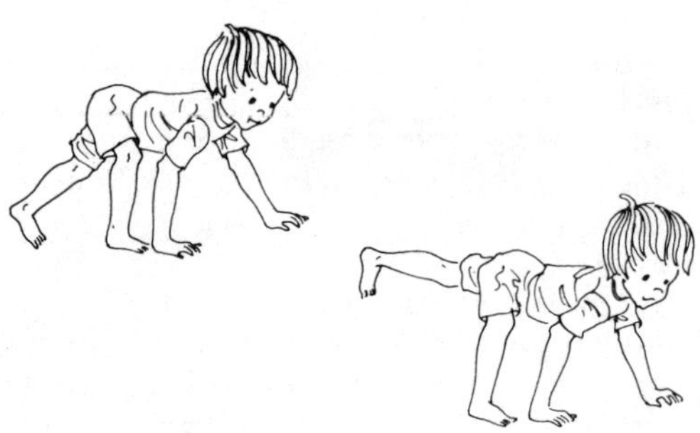

MOVEMENT INTERACTION CHALLENGES

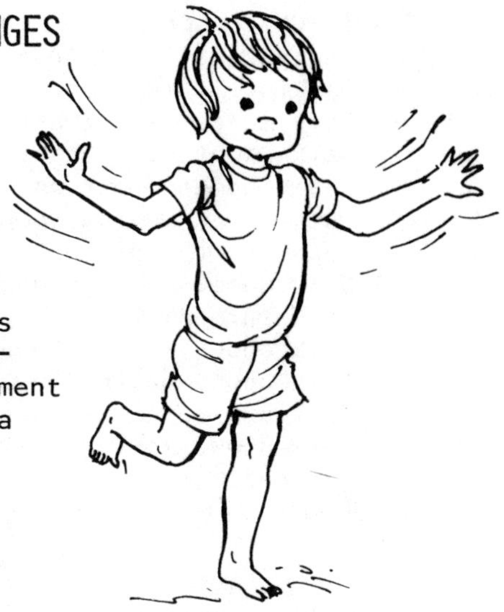

PERFORMANCE OBJECTIVES

By performing the following challenges, student demonstrates movement security within his or her own physical self (self-expression), ability to communicate and relate through movement with another person, and the ability to relate securely to a group of persons through movement experiences.

EQUIPMENT

None.

GENERAL INFORMATION

Movement can take place by oneself, with a partner, or relating to a group of persons. The concepts of self-partner-group are traditional and basic to all movement experiences. Once the child feels secure with movement within oneself, it becomes much easier to relate to another person (or partner), and finally, to groups of people. This interaction through movement can be verbal or non-verbal communication. The challenges presented in this section are designed to be non-verbal communication.

FOCUS ON SELF

Challenges in this part allow the student to focus on his or her own self so that he or she will be able to confidently say: "I can do many things successfully with my body", and "I can move and control my physical self".

STATIC CHALLENGES

These tasks emphasize static (in place) balance using axial (non-locomotor) movements.

1) Balance on 2 body parts; 3 body parts; 4 body parts, etc.
2) Balance on one foot; move very low on one foot; very high; etc.
3) Fly (flap wings) like a bird while balancing on one foot.
4) Make a complete turn on one foot without losing your balance.
5) Bend and unbend one body part; 2 parts; 3 parts; etc.
6) Twist one body part; 2 body parts, 3 body parts; etc.
7) Twist your body into the shape of a pretzel.
8) Shake one body part; 2 body parts; 3 body parts; etc.
9) Shake your whole body like a dust mop.
10) Stretch your body out like a rubber band.
11) Curl and uncurl your body like a cat.
12) Pose like different sports participants that I call out: a) golfer; b) swimmer; c) baseball player; etc.
13) On my signal (whistle, hand clap, etc.) change quickly to different athletic poses. Use your imagination!
14) Model clothes (pose) for the different seasons or weather conditions which I call out: a) Winter; b) Summer (beach); c) Fall; d) rainy weather; etc.
15) Pose like the: a) Strongest person in the world; b) Funniest person in the world; c) Saddest person in the world; and d) Scariest person in the world; etc.

DYNAMIC CHALLENGES

These tasks allow a transition from focus on self to a partner. Locomotion in the form of walking is the vehicle of communication along with facial expressions.

1) Walk in different directions looking for large spaces to move into.
2) Walk about continually moving towards someone, but make a sharp turn away just before reaching each person. Show no recognition--look through the person.
3) Walk about moving towards someone whose "eye you catch", but jump and turn just before reaching the person. Continue to walk, jump and turn, etc.
4) Walk about moving towards different persons, but try to frighten the person, (no sound) then turn away.
5) Walk about moving towards someone whose "eye you catch", smile warmly, and turn away.
6) Walk about moving towards someone, shake hands warmly, and move on to another person. Continue to warmly greet each person (no sound).
7) Walk about moving towards someone, smile, shake hands, and keep this person as your partner.

RELATING TO PARTNER

Challenges in this part allow the student to focus on partner relationships so the student will be able to confidently say: "I can move cooperatively with another person"; and "We can work successfully together to solve movement problems".

HIGH WIRE CHALLENGES (CIRCUS THEME)

Students imagine that they are walking on a high wire as in a circus.

1) Each partner will start from opposite ends of the high wire. Walk towards each other using arms to adjust balance. Remember you are on a high wire with balance very difficult to maintain. When you reach each other at the center, turn and walk back to your starting point.
2) Walk forward on high wire towards your partner, pass in the center by assisting each other without losing balance and walk to opposite end.
3) Walk forward on high wire towards your partner and when reaching each other in the center, find a way of passing each other without touching and without losing balance. You must work cooperatively!
4) One partner will carry a long balance pole and the other person will not have a pole. Walk towards each other and at the center, the partner without the pole begins losing balance. This person grabs onto his or her partner's pole. Together they struggle to maintain balance while holding the pole. Cooperatively they solve the problem and make it back to one end.

MIRROR IMAGE CHALLENGES

1) Close eyes, move slowly about reaching out with finger tips until touching someone. This person is your new partner.
2) With eyes open and without touching, one partner will create slow movements with hands and arms. Partner will mirror these movements as if looking into a mirror. Reverse roles.
3) Partners touch fingertips of both hands and move hands in various patterns. Try to feel which partner is the leader, but do not dominate your partner.
4) Close eyes and repeat same activity as in #2 above. Work cooperatively!

MISCELLANEOUS CHALLENGES (VARIOUS THEMES)

1) *Lifting Weights* - One partner is lifting weights, but cannot get weights overhead. Partner comes to this person's rescue and together they struggle to lift weights overhead with arms finally extended. Reverse roles.

2) *Pumping Up Ball* - One partner has air pump and pumps air into flat ball (other partner on the ground). After fully inflating ball, partner bounces ball (other partner) up and down. Reverse roles.
3) *Blowing Up Balloon* - One partner will blow air into balloon (other partner). After balloon is fully inflated, let the air out. Balloon sizzles to the ground. Reverse roles.
4) *Sculpturing* - One partner is the artist (sculptor) and forms clay (partner) into an art work. Move partner's body parts into various positions to form final masterpiece. Reverse roles.

RELATING TO GROUP

Challenges in this part allow the student to focus on group relationships so that the student will be able to confidently say: "I can move in cooperation and coordination with a group of people"; and "All of us can move and solve movement problems successfully together".

CHAIN CHALLENGES
1) Move about space, "catch the eye" of another person, and with facial expressions welcome this person as your new partner.
2) With your new partner join one hand, and close eyes. Move carefully about until joining hands with another set of partners to form a "chain" of 4 people.
3) With your group (chain) of 4, weave in and out under arms and tie selves into a knot. Now untie the knot.
4) Build a bridge over water with all 4 members of your group connected together to form the bridge.
5) Form a circle (standing) with your group of 4, joining hands. Working cooperatively, place your circle in a variety of balanced positions. Each time I signal, change your positions or poses without releasing hands.
6) Connect your group with another group to form a chain (group) of 8 people.
7) Weave in and out under arms to form a figure, and then unweave.

MACHINE CHALLENGES
1) Construct a machine with one person in your group of 8 becoming the first part. Each person in turn will add on to the machine to become additional parts.
2) On my signal quickly build a new machine never before created.
3) I will now turn on the power switch. The machine parts will begin to move in total coordination.
4) Show me how your machine can move to the rhythm of the music I will play. (Select appropriate music.)

TUG-A-WAR CHALLENGES
1) With your group of 8 form a straight line behind a leader. Move your group so that your leader is facing the leader of another group of 8.
2) You are now going to participate in a Tug-A-War (rope pulling) contest. Pick up the rope and space yourself on the rope so that you can use all your strength to pull with.
3) To win the contest you must pull *all* of the opposing group members over the center line which divides your 2 groups. Are you in a balanced and strong pulling position ready to begin?
4) On my signal to begin, show me how you can work cooperatively with the opposing group. Each group almost pulls the opposite group over the center line, but never quite succeeds. Both groups will finally collapse with exhaustion. Be careful not to collapse on top of your group members!

BALL CHALLENGES

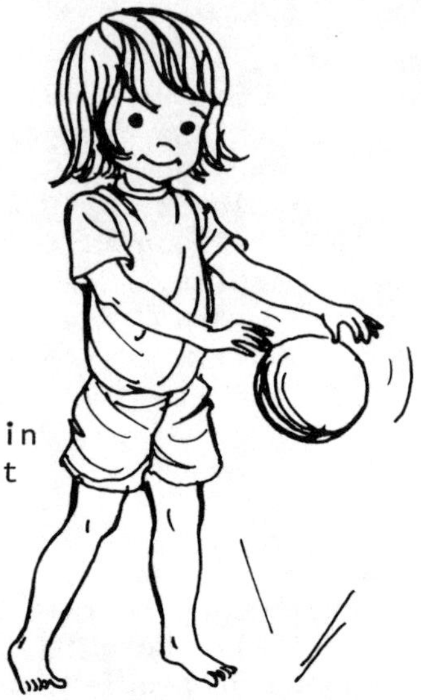

PERFORMANCE OBJECTIVES

By performing the following challenges, student demonstrates skill in handling a ball, improvement in knowledge of body parts, improvement in laterality, and development of hand-eye coordination.

EQUIPMENT

Classroom set of balls.

GENERAL INFORMATION

Each of the following ball handling lessons is easy to organize, and is listed in probable order of introduction. It must be stressed that the most effective way to carry out the lessons is to have each child in possession of a ball following the teacher's actions or directions. A 7 inch diameter or similar size rubber ball is best for these lessons.

A good starting point for all lessons is to have each child in the class holding a ball on top of his or her head with both hands. Encourage the students to allow adequate space between themselves. Inform the students that any time they hear the whistle blow, they are to stop, put the ball on top of their heads, look and listen for directions. For best control over the ball encourage the students to use finger tips in all ball-handling. *The key to success of this program is that every student has a ball to work with!!*

BODY CHALLENGES

1) Start the lesson by having the students roll the ball over and around all parts of the body calling out the names of body parts as they go. For example, start the ball rolling forward over forehead, eyebrows, nose, mouth, chin, neck, chest, stomach, down the right leg, right thigh, right knee, right ankle, right toe, to back of the right knee, etc. Stress keeping the ball always in contact with the body.
2) Ask the students to move the ball and place it against their left ears, then back to the top of their heads. Progress through the shoulders, rib-cage, hips, knees, toes, etc., all on one side of the body. Ask each student to call out "left ear", "left shoulder", "left knee", etc., as you progress.
3) Go to the opposite side of the body in the same manner as in #2 above.
4) Start mixing the commands, first to the left, then to the right. As you progress with this activity you will find that many students who had difficulty in the beginning are gradually becoming more familiar with all their body parts as well as the left and right sides of their bodies.

DROP AND CATCH CHALLENGES

This lesson will involve a series of drop and catch activities that will once again place emphasis on the student's body parts, and knowledge of left and right. Hand-eye coordination will be refined.

1) Holding the ball on top of your head, take one step back, let the ball roll forward, bounce once, and catch it with both hands.
2) Hold ball alternately on right, then left eye, step back, drop and catch it with both hands.

3) Repeat this type of activity using different body parts always stressing the right and left to the students.
4) Holding the ball on top of the head once again, have the students step forward, turn to their left, drop and catch the ball, then to their right, drop and catch the ball.
5) Ask students to put the ball underneath the right armpit and then the left armpit, lift arm from the side, let the ball bounce and try to catch it with one hand, either right or left.
6) Hold the ball high in the right hand (arm extended), release the ball, let it bounce, and catch it.
7) Repeat above task using the left hand.

SPECIAL NOTATION - During the above lessons on Body Challenges and Drop And Catch Challenges, you will find that each student will take great delight in calling to your attention that they were successful. In fact, the students tend to react this way through all of these activities and they should be given verbal "pats on the back" for accomplishment whenever possible. You will notice many students dropping the ball often as you progress which indicates that these students need more of this kind of ball activity prior to working with others in throw and catch situations. This type of activity can be quite challenging as you have the students gradually attempt more difficult maneuvers such as moving the ball with only one hand around opposite arms, behind the head, neck, back, over the buttocks, etc., but the students will try everything if they have a ball. The fact that they have trouble on some of the activities will not embarrass them as you will find that the students are quite unaware of what others are doing or failing to do!

√TRICK CHALLENGES

This lesson consists of trying as many different tricks with the ball as possible.

1) Ask the students if they can hold the ball with the backs of their hands, then back of right hand and palm of the left hand, etc.
2) Ask students to hold ball with only 4 fingers, then 3, 2, and finally with only one finger of each hand.
3) Hold the ball with the fingers of both hands. See how quickly you can make the ball turn forwards and backwards using the finger tips to maneuver the ball.
4) Try to quickly pass the ball from hand to hand around your waist. Do not touch the ball to your body. Now change directions.
5) Try this same type of task passing the ball from hand to hand between and around your knees.
6) Place the ball between the thighs of the legs, jump, spread the legs letting the ball bounce, then try to catch it with the hands. Do this same thing placing the ball between the knees, calves, and ankles. (Each time the ball is placed closer to the ground the student must jump a little higher in order to get a good bounce from the ball.)
7) Ask the students to place the ball on their stomachs, then roll it around to their backs. Then have them roll it down over the buttocks and legs until they are holding it between their legs about knee high. Then ask them to flip the ball into the air with their hands, then bringing their hands in front of their body to catch it.
8) Ask the students to place the ball behind their necks and lean slightly forward. Then tell them to let go of the ball and try to quickly put their hands behind their backs palms up, and attempt to catch the ball as it rolls down their backs.

√BASIC EXPLORATION CHALLENGES

Teacher should suggest various challenges to the students. (Can you do this...?, Who can..?, Show me how you can..., etc.) *Each child has a ball!*

1) Bounce and catch the ball with 2 hands.
2) Bounce, clap hands, and catch.
3) Bounce under each leg and catch.
4) Roll ball, run and field it.

5) Toss above head, let bounce and catch.
6) Toss above head, let bounce, turn and catch.
7) Toss above head and catch.
8) Toss above head, clap hands, and catch.
9) Toss ball from hand to hand.
10) Toss ball into the air, jump off ground and catch it.
11) Run, toss ball in air and catch.
12) Use finger tips and tap (volley) ball in the air 2 times and catch it, then 3 times, etc.
13) Jump over ball forward and backward.
14) Place ball between knees and hop like a kangaroo.
15) Use the sides of your feet to dribble (control) the ball in your immediate space.

√ THROWING AND CATCHING PARTNER CHALLENGES

1) Underhand toss to partner using 2 hands.
2) Underhand toss to partner using one hand.
3) Overhand toss to partner using 2 hands (chest pass).
4) Overhand toss to partner using one hand.
5) Bounce pass to partner using 2 hands.
6) Bounce pass to partner using one hand.
7) Underhand high toss to partner.
8) Overhead pass to partners using 2 hands.

√ HAND DRIBBLING CHALLENGES

1) Bounce and catch using 2 hands.
2) 2 hand dribble (continuously bouncing ball without catching).
3) Preferred hand dribble in place.
4) Dribble low and high in place.
5) Least preferred hand dribble in place.
6) Walk and dribble using preferred hand.
7) Walk and dribble using least preferred hand.
8) Changing hands dribble in place.
9) Walk and dribble while changing hands.
10) Run and dribble using either hand.
11) Run and dribble with eyes off ball.
12) Stop and go dribbling. (Teacher uses hand signals indicating when to stop and go.)
13) Dribble in small circles, then larger circles.
14) Dribble in different directions looking for large openings.

HAND STRIKING CHALLENGES

1) Drop ball and hit to partner with 2 hands using fingers.
2) Drop ball and hit to partner with one hand using fingers.
3) Sock ball from hand with a bounce to partner.
4) Drop and serve (hit) ball to partner by using closed hand.
5) Serve (hit) ball out of hand to partner by using closed hand.
6) Hit ball back and forth with partner (no catching, using only open hands). (Note: You may wish to have students hit back and forth over a line.)

ROLLING AND THROWING CHALLENGES

Use bowling pins as targets and have at least 6 drill stations going at once. 3 chalk restraining lines should be marked off at various distances opposite each pin. 5 students are assigned to each group. One catcher, one performer, and 3 in line waiting to perform. Each performer has 3 trials, in order, and then rotates to catcher. Catcher then rotates to end of waiting line. If pin is knocked over from first line, performer moves to 2nd line for next trial. Goal of each performer is to knock the pin down from each of the 3 lines.

1) Underhand bowling or ball rolling using 2 hands.
2) Underhand bowling or ball rolling using one hand.
3) Underhand pitch or toss using one hand.
4) Overhand pitch or throw using one hand.

KICKING CHALLENGES – Spring

Set up at least 4 drill stations having 5 or 6 students at each station. Each group of students will have a kicker, pitcher, fielder, and waiting line to kick. The kicker, pitcher, and fielder are in a straight line formation spaced equal distance apart. Use kick balls.

1) Kicking a stationary ball. A short run of 3 or 4 steps up to ball may be used by kicker. Pitcher fields the ball or is passed the ball from the fielder. Pitcher then runs in with the ball, hands it to the next kicker and goes to the end of the waiting line. Fielder rotates to the pitching position, and kicker goes to the fielder's position.
2) Kicking a rolling ball. Same procedure as in #1 above except pitcher rolls ball to kicker and fielder has ball when he or she rotates to pitcher's position.
3) Target kicking. Use a pin and 3 chalk restraining lines at various distances from the pin. Each kicker has 3 trials, and moves back a line each time the pin is knocked over.

FOOT DRIBBLING AND PASSING CHALLENGES Spring

Use kick balls and line up students in 4 or 6 relay formation groups. Explain to students that dribbling and heeling skills are necessary to play soccer type games.

1) Dribble ball using sides of both feet down to a goal line and back.
2) Dribble ball using sides of both feet around obstacles. Use bases or pins as obstacles.
3) Dribble and pass with partner using inside and outside of feet. 2 relay lines work together with students passing the ball back and forth as they move it down the field.
4) Stationary passing. Students form a square and pass the ball from player to player around the square. Students should be shown how to trap (stop) ball using their heel.

BASKET SHOOTING CHALLENGES

Set up 4 to 8 shooting stations using large waste paper baskets as the target and rubber utility balls (preferaby 8 inch size) to shoot with 3 chalk restraining lines should be marked off at various distances opposite each basket. Students are assigned to each station: one catcher, one shooter, and 2 or 3 in line waiting their turn. Each shooter has 3 trials in order and then rotates to catcher. Catcher then rotates to end of waiting line. If a basket is made from the first line, shooter moves to 2nd line for next trial. Goal of each shooter is to make a basket from each of the 3 restraining lines.

1) Underhand shooting. Use both hands under ball.
2) Overhand set shot. Use both hands in applying equal force to push the ball forward from the chest area.
3) Overhand one-handed set shot. Use one hand to support the ball, and the other hand to push it for a basket.
4) Basket bounce shooting. Use both hands to push ball down so that it bounces into the basket. This drill would be used mainly to provide more variation.

Note: If enough regular basketball baskets are available at a low enough height to allow students to be successful, this activity could then be used with the regular baskets. This is not usually the case with younger children.

ROPE CHALLENGES

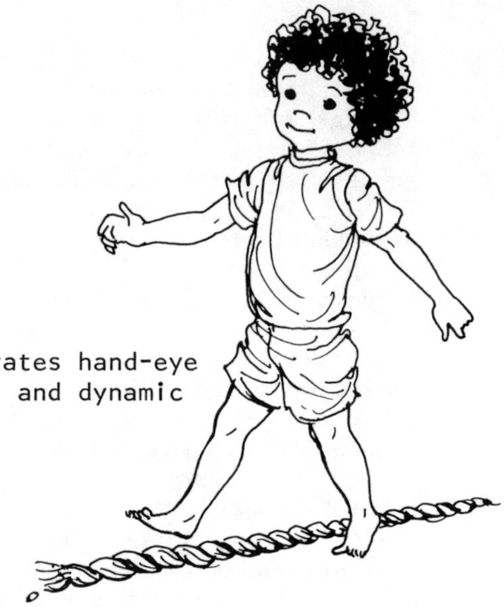

PERFORMANCE OBJECTIVES

By performing the following challenges, student demonstrates hand-eye and foot-eye coordination, rhythm, agility, flexibility, and dynamic balance.

EQUIPMENT

Classroom set of jump ropes.

GENERAL INFORMATION

The following lessons with jump ropes represent a slight departure from the use of ropes in the traditional manner. It must be stressed that in each of these lessons it is most desirable that each student have a rope. Ropes are approximately 7 feet long. Each student reacts to the directed challenge according to his or her own interpretation of the problem. To begin the following challenges, each student should place his or her rope on the ground in a straight line. The student stands at one end of the rope facing the instructor.

ROPE WALKING CHALLENGES

1) Walk around the rope without touching it.
2) Straddle the rope with one foot on each side and walk down to the end and back without turning around.
3) Walk beside the rope on the right side, step over at the end, and walk backward on the left side.
4) Walk around the rope using a toe-heel balance walk.
5) Walk the length of the rope forward and back to starting position, balancing on top of the rope.
6) Stand at the end of the rope with feet straddling the rope, and walk forward using a criss-cross step (left leg over right, right over left, etc.). Move forward down and back.
7) Using a criss-cross walk, move backwards down to the end of the rope and back.

ROPE JUMPING AND HOPPING CHALLENGES

1) With feet straddling the rope, jump down and back without turning around.
2) Standing to the right of the rope, jump down with both feet together, jump across the rope at the end, and jump backward on the left side to starting position.
3) Standing at the end of the rope with feet together on the right side, jump back and forth, right to left and left to right down the rope and back to starting position.
4) Standing at the end of the rope, hop down on the right foot, hop across the rope, and hop back on the left foot. (This pattern can be changed many times using various combinations of left and right.)
5) Standing at the end of the rope, balance on the right foot, and hop right side to left side, etc., hopping back and forth down to the end and back.
6) Stand to the right of the rope at the end, turn and face the rope. With both feet together, jump over the rope and back again, moving from left to right down the rope and back to starting position. (Student is facing the rope and jumping forward and backward over the rope.)
7) Stand to the right of the rope as in Challenge #6, turn and face the rope. Hop over

the rope forward and backward on the right foot, moving from left to right down the rope and back.

8) Straddle the rope with both feet, then jump into the air and cross left foot over right foot so that the feet continue to straddle the rope, only now they are in a crossed position. Next, jump into the air and uncross the feet but land straddling the rope. Continue this same pattern.

√ROPE ANIMAL WALK CHALLENGES

1) Straddle the rope in a bear walk position (hands and feet on the ground) and walk down and back moving the opposite hand and foot in coordination.
2) Straddle the rope in a bear walk position and walk down and back moving the left hand and left foot only, and then the right hand and right foot only.
3) Straddle the rope in a bear walk position. Walk down and back moving both hands first, then both feet.
4) Straddle the rope in a crab walk position (hands and feet on the ground with stomach up). Walk down and back moving the opposite hand and foot.
5) Straddle the rope in a crab walk position. Walk down and back moving the left hand and left foot, then the right hand and the right foot.
6) Straddle the rope in a bear walk position. Walk down and back criss-crossing the left hand over the right hand and right hand over the left hand.
7) Straddle the rope in a bear walk position. Walk down and back criss-crossing the left foot over the right foot and the right foot over the left foot.
8) Straddle the rope in a bear walk position. Walk down and back criss-crossing both the feet and the hands at the same time. (A tough challenge!)

√ROPE CIRCLE CHALLENGES

Ask students to make a circle with their ropes on the floor.

1) Who can jump to the center of his or her circle and out again without touching the rope?
2) Can you jump forwards and backwards, in and out, of your circle?
3) Now, try jumping sidewards, in and out of your circle.
4) Show me how you can jump completely over your circle and land softly on the other side. Use your arms to help lift your body.
5) Can you hop around your rope circle on one foot? Now change direction and hop on the other foot.
6) Who can hop into the center of his or her circle on one foot, then hop out on the opposite foot?
7) Can you move around your circle with:
   a) One hand touching the floor inside.
   b) One foot touching the floor inside.
   c) Two hands touching inside the circle.
   d) One hand and one foot touching inside.
   e) Discover other ways of moving around your circle.
8) Can you build a bridge completely over your circle by using your hands and feet to balance on?
9) Can you make your bridge move around the circle?
10) As a final challenge, show me how you can jump from circle to circle around in our space without any collisions. "Freeze" on my signal.

√ROPE LETTER AND NUMBER CHALLENGES

1) Ask students to form letters with their ropes such as the letter (small) "c". Ask them to stand at the base of their ropes and decide if the open end points to their left or right.
2) Ask the students to form the letter (small) "b" with their ropes. Ask if the loop at the bottom of the letter faces to their left or right.
3) Repeat Challenge #2 above with the small letter "d".

4) Ask the students to form letters such as a small "q" and a small "p". Again ask them if the letter faces to their left or right.
5) Ask students to make the same letters using their bodies over the rope position.
6) If the student has 2 ropes, the above activities can be achieved with a great number of the letters in the English alphabet.
7) Ask students to form numbers with their ropes such as the number "2". Ask them to stand at the bottom of their ropes and decide if the open end faces to the left or right.
8) Numbers such as "6" or "9" are also good numbers to try. Numbers such as "5" and "8" are even more challenging.
9) You can ask the students to walk, jump, hop, etc., the length of the rope while it is in the form of a letter or number. (It is felt this increases the student's chance of achieving basic directionality.)
10) Try some simple math problems. Have students give answers using their ropes. (Example, 3 + 4 = ?)

ROPE TURNING AND JUMPING CHALLENGES

1) Student grasps both ends of rope in right hand.
    a) Student turns rope on right side of body while allowing the rope to hit the ground with each complete turn.
    b) Student turns rope, and jumps in rhythm with each turn. Jump is timed with rope hitting the ground.
2) Student repeats same action as in #1 above but uses left hand for holding rope.
3) Student has one rope in each hand. (Have children pair off and take turns, if lacking ropes.)
    a) Keeping elbows in close to hips, student turns both ropes at once in rhythm.
    b) Student turns both ropes at once, and jumps in rhythm with the turning ropes. Jump is timed with ropes hitting ground.
4) Student holds rope just in front of his or her feet with one end of the rope held in each hand.
    a) With feet together, student jumps back and forth over the rope without moving it.
    b) Repeat above with a hop on the left foot and then a hop on the right foot.
5) Student holds rope in front of feet and swings it slowly back and forth under feet. Student then attempts to jump it with both feet together, forward and backward.
6) Student holds end of rope in each hand and places the center of the rope touching ground a few feet out in front of his or her body. Student then drags rope towards feet and jumps it just before it reaches his or her toes.
7) Student is asked to hold rope behind heels to be in starting position to jump rope. Student then swings rope over head so that it hits the ground several feet in front of body, and drags rope to feet and jumps it.
8) Student repeats item #7, but turns rope faster and attempts one regular jump.
    a) Student next trys for 2 jumps in succession, then 3, 4, etc.
    b) Students still having difficulty with releasing both feet off the ground in rhythm, or in turning the rope, will have to go back and practice activity drills which stress those skills.

Note: Teacher must decide how much repetition is needed on each of the 8 listed drills. Teacher may wish to eliminate some of these drills, or change their order of progression depending on the ability level and interest of the students.

HOOP CHALLENGES

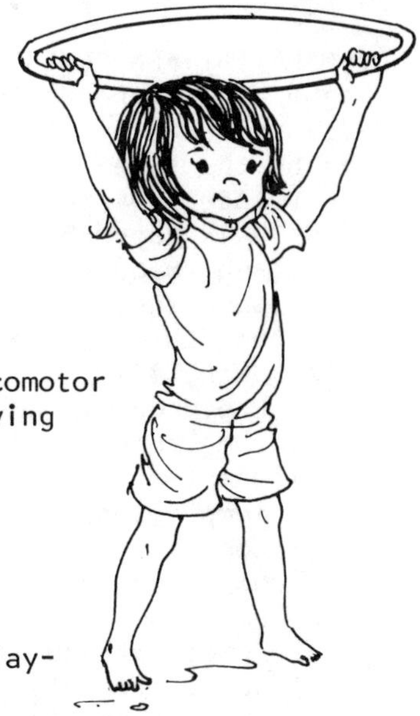

PERFORMANCE OBJECTIVES

By performing the following challenges, student demonstrates locomotor skills, manipulation skills, spatial awareness, and problem solving ability.

EQUIPMENT

Classroom set of hoops.

GENERAL INFORMATION

1) Large area needed with hard surface like a cafeteria, gym, playground, or hard top.
2) Background music is helpful, but certainly not essential.
3) Best to have one hoop per student (minimum of one hoop for 2 students).
4) Students are told to select a "home" site within a given area and stand inside their home (hoop).
5) Teacher then proceeds with selected hoop lesson. Below are listed 5 suggested lesson plans which may be used. These plans, of course, are only scratching the surface of ideas.

√ EXPLORATION CHALLENGES

1) Can you reach down and pick up the hoop without bending your knees?
2) How high up can you stretch with the hoop held in both hands?
3) Can you hold hoop above your head and drop it so that it hits the ground without touching your body?
4) Can you balance your weight on one foot within your hoop and lean forward from the waist?
5) Can you spin the hoop and keep it going like an egg beater?
6) Can you jump in and out of the hoop while holding it on end?
7) Can you use the hoop like a jump rope?
8) Being careful not to bump into anyone, can you roll your hoop and keep it from falling over?
9) While your hoop is rolling, can you run around it without touching it?
10) Can you move through your hoop while it is rolling?
11) Who can throw the hoop in the air and catch it before it lands? Can you throw it still higher and catch it?
12) How can you throw the hoop on the floor so that it will roll back to you?
13) Can you climb in and out and around your own hoop?
14) What other exciting things can you do with your hoop?

Have students pick partners to perform the remaining Exploration Challenges.

15) Can you exchange hoops with a partner by rolling them back and forth? Do it in rhythm!
16) Who can jump into a hoop held low to the floor by your partner? Now let your partner try it while you hold the hoop.
17) As your partner holds *both* hoops in different positions, let's see who can go through *both* hoops without touching either hoop. Now let your partner try.
18) Using one hoop, can you toss and catch the hoop with your partner? Now try tossing and catching 2 hoops with your partner.
19) Can you catch a hoop which has been thrown by your partner on your arm? Can you spin it on this same arm?
20) What other ways can you discover to exchange hoops with your partner?

MOVEMENT PATTERN CHALLENGES

Use 6 or more hoops in each pattern. Set up at least 4 patterns, divide students evenly, and assign them to the patterns. All patterns may be the same, or each one may be different so that students can rotate from pattern to pattern.

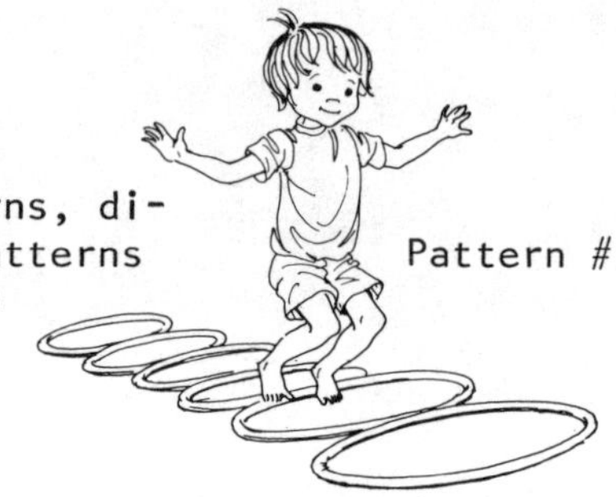

Pattern #1

1) a) Walk through the pattern.
   b) Run through the pattern.
   c) Jump through the pattern.
   d) Hop through the pattern.
2) a) Jump, jump, straddle jump, jump, jump.
   b) Hop, hop, straddle jump, hop, hop.
   c) Jump, hop, straddle jump, hop, jump.

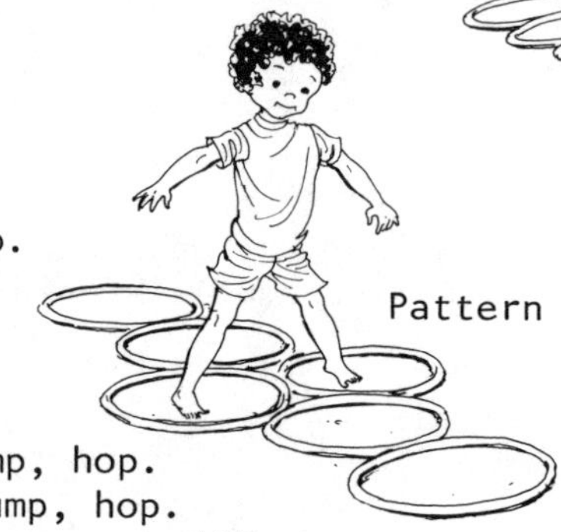

Pattern #2

3) a) Jump, straddle jump, jump, straddle jump, jump.
   b) Hop, straddle jump, hop, straddle jump, hop.
   c) Hop, straddle jump, jump, straddle jump, hop.
4) a) Left foot hop, straddle jump, right hop, straddle jump, left hop.
   b) Jump, straddle jump, right hop, straddle jump, left hop.
   c) Hop the pattern changing from left to right and back to left. (Left, left, right, right, right, left, left.)

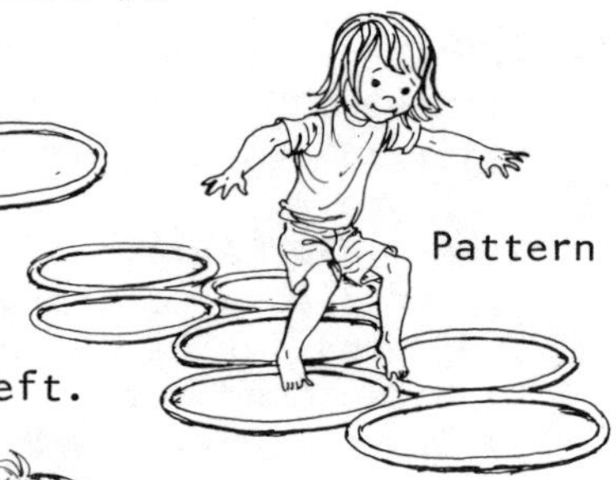

Pattern #3

BODY PARTS AND MOTION CHALLENGES

Student works in confined space of selected "home" area.

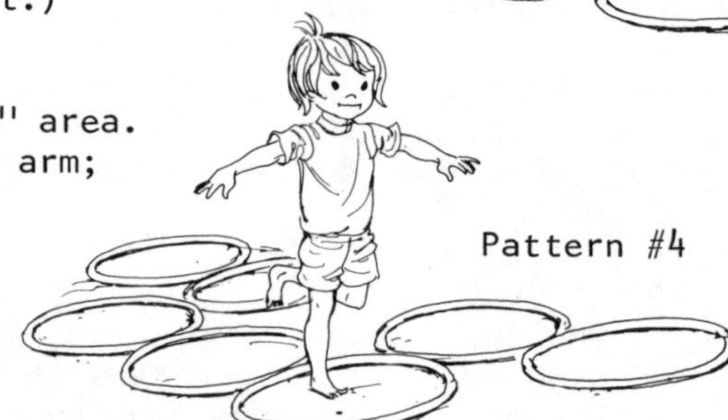

Pattern #4

1) Students are asked to move the hoop around: a) arm; b) wrist; c) elbow; d) neck; e) waist; f) leg; g) knees; and h) ankle.
2) Students attempt to move hoop from one part of the body to another. Examples: a) Down (neck to knees and waist to ankles, etc.); and b) Up (hips to shoulders and knees to hips, etc.)
3) Students use concept of force and change in levels (posture) using the hoop motion skills stressed in Challenge #1 above. Examples: a) How fast can you make the hoop go?; b) How slow can you make the hoop go?; c) Can you go from fast to slow and slow to fast?; and d) How low can you move your body and still keep the hoop moving? (Lowest would be to lie on back and move hoop around arm.)
4) Students use hoop motion skills in moving through space. Examples: a) Use above skills while moving fast or slow, etc.; and b) Create patterns singly and with partners.

ACCENT BEAT AND BASIC MOVEMENT CHALLENGES

1) Students walk around hoop and hop inside of hoop on the accent beat which can be a hand clap, drum beat, etc. (Or reverse direction on the accent beat, squat on the accent beat, etc.)
2) Students use various movement skills such as a slide, gallop, step-draw, skip, hop, etc., to move around the hoop in a definite rhythm.
3) Students perform various types of animal walks around the hoop such as a bear walk, kangaroo hop, elephant walk, etc. Hoop represents a cage and on an accent beat or command they must jump into the cage.
4) Students place hoops inside of a large multi-purpose game court and line up around the outside of the court. On a signal (whistle) students move around the outside of the court using movement skills designated by the instructor (marching, skipping, running, etc.). On the next signal (whistle) students must run for their "home" (hoop). Students are eliminated if they contact another student while running to their "home". Music adds greatly to this activity. Students learn spatial awareness as well as practicing movement patterns to the music.
5) Students stand inside of their "home" (hoop) and on a signal use various movement skills to find a new home. Each time the signal is given, students must quickly find a new home. On the final signal, students must arrive back at their original home.

6) Students use their own creative movement ideas to move around the hoop. Instructor gives them problems to solve. They can learn to develop several movement skills into a pattern.

BALL SKILL CHALLENGES

1) Students begin with a rubber ball 7 to 8 inches in diameter in their possession and are standing inside of their home.
2) Start with problem solving approach: Can they bounce the ball while keeping it inside the hoop? Can they toss the ball above head level and make it bounce inside of the hoop? Etc.
3) Next have students move in a pattern around the outside of the hoop while they: Bounce and catch the ball; dribble the ball; walk, toss, and catch the ball; etc.
4) Students next work with a partner using one ball between them and one hoop. One partner stands on each side of the hoop.
   a) Students bounce the ball so that it hits inside of the hoop and partner can catch it.
   b) Students bounce the ball and strike (slap) it with the fingers like in 4-square so that the ball hits once inside of the hoop. Partner catches ball and returns it with the same technique.
   c) Students bounce and slap the ball while attempting to keep it in continuous movement. They do not catch the ball!
   d) Teacher may wish to have students experiment with each student having a ball. They attempt to exchange balls with a bounce and catch without the balls contacting each other.

GAME CHALLENGES

1) *HOOP WAR (grades 5 to 8)*
   a) Select 2 teams and have teams face each other approximately 15 feet apart.
   b) Use music for stimulation (fast beat, if possible).
   c) First person in each line comes forward keeping hoop moving around the waist. Object is to knock hoop off opponent's waist while keeping own hoop going.
   d) Winning player scores one point for the team and new players come forward. If both hoops are knocked off, no points are awarded.
   e) To keep more people active at one time you can give players a number and call off several numbers at one time, or have 4 teams, and have one player from each team come out at once. Last player with hoop still going scores a point for his/her team.
2) *HOOP TAG*
   Have definite boundaries and have hoops placed within the boundary lines. Use about 1/4 as many hoops as there are students.
   a) One or 2 students are "It" (chasers) and they attempt to tag other students with one hand above the waist, or they can hold a ball and tag players with the ball.
   b) A player *cannot* be tagged while standing with both feet inside of a hoop, but only one player can be in a hoop at one time. When one player enters a hoop, any other player in that hoop must leave.
   c) A player cannot stand for over 10 seconds in a hoop.
   d) Players tagged become "poison" and must freeze where tagged. They can tag other players who come within their reach. However, they cannot move their feet.
   e) "It" cannot enter or run through the hoops. Players cannot run out of bounds. If players run out of bounds, they are penalized by having to freeze at the spot where they left the court.
   f) Last player or last 2 players caught are the winners and become the new chasers.
   g) Optional rules: Chasers can throw a ball at players and attempt to hit them below the waist with the ball. Players can be given various types of movement patterns which change throughout the game at a signal by the teacher (skip, walk, hop, etc.).

3) *MUSICAL HOOPS*

Played like musical chairs only hoops are used. Hoops can be placed in large circle formation, or scattered about inside boundary lines of a multi-purpose court on the playground.

a) Music is played and students march around the hoops placed in a large circle, or they march around boundary lines of a large game court with hoops placed inside of court.
b) When the music stops or on a signal (whistle), all the players attempt to get inside a hoop. One player to a hoop.
c) Each time players begin to march around, hoops are taken from playing area so that there are less hoops than players left in the game.
d) Players who fail to get inside a hoop on the signal are eliminated from the game.
e) Last player left is the winner.
f) Optional rules: Instead of just plain walking or marching, have students use other movement skills like sliding, skipping, etc.

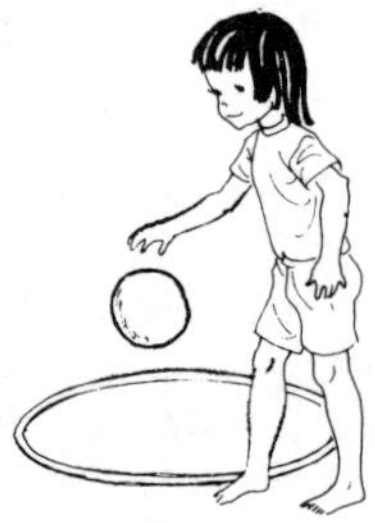

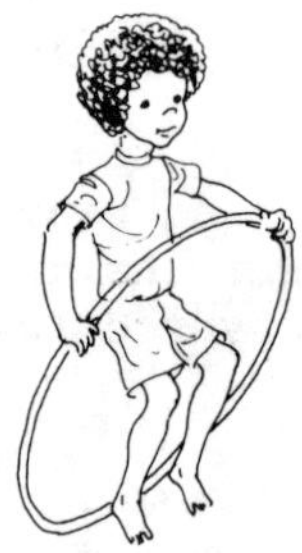

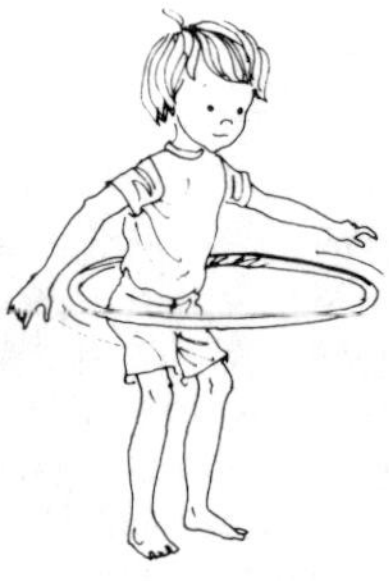

BEAN BAG CHALLENGES

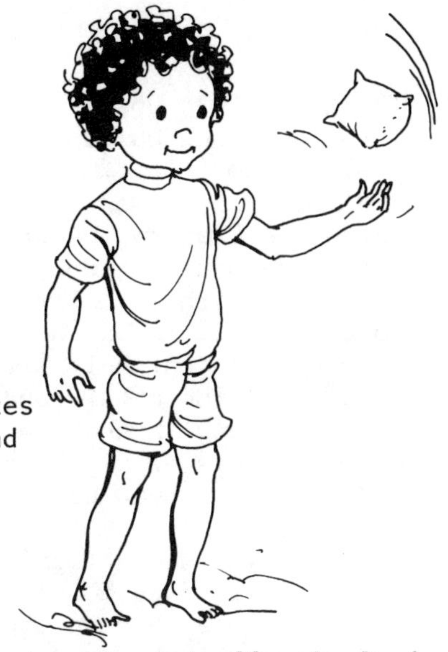

PERFORMANCE OBJECTIVES

By performing the following challenges, student demonstrates hand-eye coordination, balance, laterality, body image, and ocular pursuit skills.

EQUIPMENT

Classroom set of bean bags.

GENERAL INFORMATION

The bean bag represents an inexpensive teaching tool which can be used effectively in the physical education program to reinforce perceptual-motor abilities. It is important that enough bean bags are available so that each student has one to use. Large numbers of bean bags can be easily stored in a plastic bucket or box which is an added advantage to their use. The teacher should basically use a Movement Exploration approach when presenting challenging tasks to the students.

ORGANIZATION

1) Best to use a scatter formation with each student working within his/her own "personal" space.
2) Students may be standing, seated, kneeling or lying on their backs depending on the types of challenges used.
3) Students should work individually at first, but gradually introduce partner activities.
4) Physical and mental involvement of all students in the lesson is the key to success! Each student should have a bean bag in his/her possession for continuous active involvement.
5) The bean bag, with its softness and flatness, has definite advantages over other manipulative implements. It does not "sting" the hands, or bounce and roll away which makes it easy to use and control for hand-eye coordination tasks. In addition, it can be easily balanced on various body parts or used as an obstacle on the ground.

THROWING AND CATCHING CHALLENGES

1) Throw bean bag upward (under-arm throw) and catch it without moving feet. Emphasis on control!
   a) Catch with 2 hands.
   b) Catch with the right hand.
   c) Catch with the left hand.
   d) Alternate hands. Throw with one hand and catch with the other.
2) Flip the bean bag 1/2 turn and catch it ("turn the pancake over").
   a) Use 2 hands with palms up.
   b) Use right hand with palm up.
   c) Use left hand with palm up.
3) Perform same challenges as in Challenge #2 above but after flipping the bean bag upward, quickly turn hands (or hand) with palms down and catch bean bag on the tops of the hands (or hand).
4) Toss bean bag back and forth across body from hand to hand.
   a) After success with simple toss, try eye tracking bean bag without moving head.
   b) Try keeping bean bag in "flat" position ("flat bread") and pass back and forth using small, quick exchanges.
   c) Using a wider distance, toss bean bag across body with rhythmical swing from hand to hand.

5) Throw bean bag upward above head and jump to catch it at the highest possible point.
6) Throw bean bag up above head, clap hands and catch it.
   a) Can you clap 2 times and catch it?
   b) How many times can you clap your hands before catching the bean bag?
7) Throw the bean bag upward and forward, then run forward and catch it.
8) Place the bean bag on your foot (or instep), then swing the bean bag upward from your foot and catch it. Try it on each foot.
9) Hold bean bag in one hand with arm extended straight up above head level. Release bean bag and catch it with the same hand before it reaches the floor. Try the same task using the other hand.
10) Hold bean bag in one hand above head level and have opposite hand and arm hanging downward at the side of the body. Release bean bag and reach across the body (mid-line) and catch the bean bag with the opposite hand. Try the same task by reversing hand positions.
11) Look at stationary focal (fixation) point and try to throw and catch the bean bag while keeping eyes focused on the fixation point.
12) Place the bean bag on top of your head, then tilt your head forward and catch the bean bag using both hands.
   a) Can you catch it using a knee or knees?
   b) Can you catch it with your feet?
13) Toss the bean bag upward, then close your eyes and catch it.
14) Try tossing and catching bean bag while in other body positions such as kneeling, sitting, or lying on back. While in these different positions, try the following tasks:
   a) Toss bean bag back and forth from hand to hand.
   b) Flip the pancake (bean bag) over 1/2 turn. Also try a full turn.
   c) Throw the bean bag up fairly high, stand quickly and catch it.
15) Toss the bean bag up above head level and attempt to catch it on top of your head without the use of your hands.
16) Throw the bean bag at a rebound net and catch it. Set up several nets, if available, or use one net as a station activity.

THROWING CHALLENGES

1) Throw the bean bag *over* a designated "goal" line, then run and retrieve it. Try throwing with each hand.
2) Throw the bean bag *at or through* a target. Try each hand.
   a) Throw at a target or spot on the wall.
   b) Throw at a rebound net.
   c) Throw the bean bag through a hoop or tire suspended or held in the air.
3) Toss the bean bag *into* a target. Try each hand.
   a) Toss the bean bag into a bike tire or hoop. Start close and after each success, increase the distance.
   b) Set up a series of tires or hoops, and attempt to toss one bean bag into each target.
   c) Use basic geometric shapes (circles, squares, triangles, etc.) either painted or drawn on playground, or else made from plywood or cardboard, and toss bean bags into designated shapes. Try matching colors also.

Note: On throwing action, emphasize a cross-lateral movement. Student steps forward to transfer weight into throw, using opposite foot from throwing hand.

LOCOMOTOR CHALLENGES

1) Place your bean bag on the floor.
   a) Can you jump over it? (Forward, sideward, and backward.)
   b) Try hopping over it on your right foot and then your left foot. Can you catch your weight on each foot without losing your balance?
   c) Can you run and leap over your bean bag?
   d) How quickly can you move around your bean bag?
   e) Can you creep around your bean bag?

f) Show me how many different parts of your body you can move the bean bag with. Try elbows, feet, head, etc.

2) Place the bean bag between the feet and jump forward. Now try jumping in a small circle.
3) With the bean bag between feet or ankles, jump into the air, release the bean bag and catch it with the hands.
4) Hold the bean bag between knees and jump like a kangaroo.
5) Walk forward and backward while balancing a bean bag on your head.
6) Try balancing the bean bag on other body parts (shoulder, foot, chin, etc.) and walking.
7) Hop on one foot while balancing the bean bag on the opposite foot. Also try the opposite knee.
8) Move like a crab (inverted body position) and balance bean bag on your stomach area.

AGILITY CHALLENGES

1) Pass the bean bag around the waist exchanging it from hand to hand behind your back and in front of your body. On a signal (whistle) change direction of the movement.
2) Rotate the bean bag around your head exchanging from hand to hand behind the neck and under the chin. Change direction on the whistle signal.
3) Pass the bean bag from hand to hand in a figure-eight pattern in and out and around the legs at knee level. Stop movement on a whistle signal and quickly change direction of the movement.
4) Place the bean bag on your head while standing with your feet apart. Bend backwards so that the bag falls off your head. Now bend forward, reach between your legs and pick up the bean bag. Quickly repeat the entire pattern.

STATIC BALANCE CHALLENGES

1) Balance the bean bag on various body parts: head, chin, shoulder, knee, foot, wrist, elbow, etc.
2) Balance the bean bag on your head, sit down and stand up without dropping the bean bag.
3) Balance the bean bag on your head, rotate your head in as large a circle as possible without moving your feet or dropping your bean bag.
4) Place your bean bag on the floor.
    a) Build a bridge over it using 4 body parts touching the floor to balance.
    b) Build a bridge over the bean bag using 3 body parts; 5 body parts; etc.
    c) Make a long bridge, a high bridge, a low bridge, a wide bridge, a draw bridge, etc.
5) Balance a bean bag on your foot (instep). Now swing your leg forward and back keeping the bean bag in place. Try the opposite foot.
6) Hold the bean bag in one hand with your arm extended forward. Kick each leg up (one at a time), and touch the hand holding the bean bag. Change hands and perform the same task.
7) Sit with legs straight and balance (hold) the bean bag between your feet. Lift your legs upward while rocking backward and touch the bean bag to the floor in back of your head. Now rock back to sitting position without dropping the bean bag.
8) Try the same task as in Challenge #7 above, but place the bean bag on the floor in back of your head and attempt to pick it up with your feet and return to a sitting position.

PARTNER CHALLENGES

1) Throw the bean bag to a partner using an underarm toss. Partner catches it using both hands.
2) Same as Challenge #1 above, only use an overhand throw.
3) Toss the bean bag high to a partner. Then toss gradually lower with each throw.
4) Throw and catch with a partner, alternating hands. Throw with one hand, catch with the other, etc.
5) Throw bean bag to a partner and just as the throw is beginning call out "right", "left", or "both". Partner must catch the bean bag with the designated hand or hands.
6) Toss and exchange bean bags in the air with your partner. Both throw at the same time.
7) Try to move around the available space with your partner and exchange bean bags.

8) Partners stand back to back with feet apart and pass one bean bag around their bodies exchanging it from hand to hand. Partners attempt to move farther apart without stopping movement pattern.
9) Same as Challenge #8 above, only bean bag must travel in a figure-eight pattern around bodies, in and out and around legs.
10) Partners engage in a bean bag grab contest by sitting and facing each other with bean bag placed on the floor between them. Instructor calls out "right", "left", or "both". Partners must have hands on hips and respond with correct hand or hands. Object is to see which partner can grab the bean bag first using the designated hand or hands.

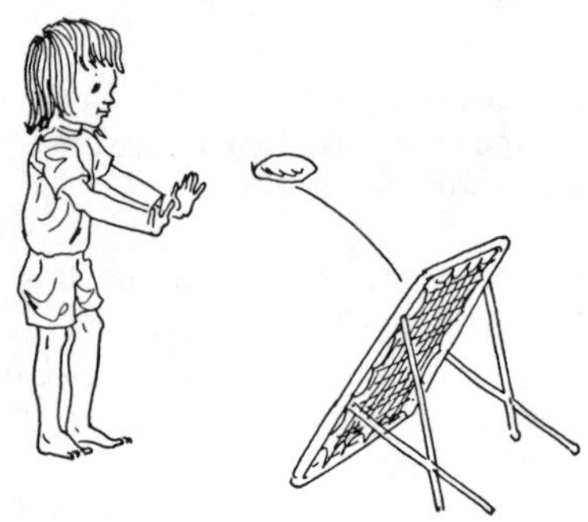

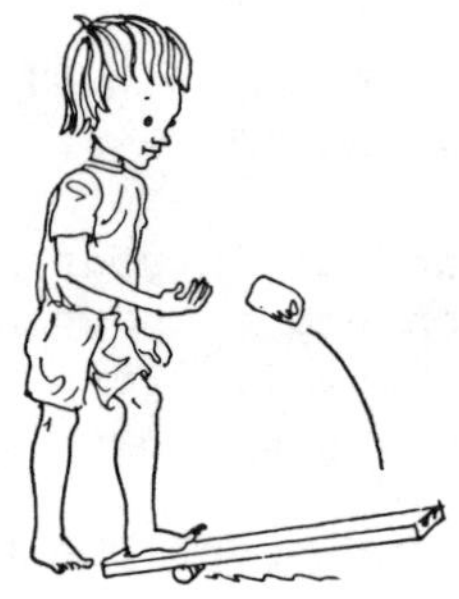

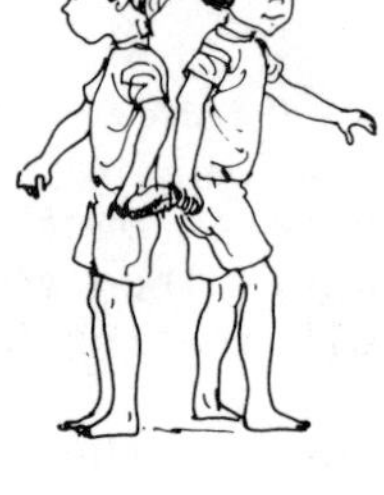

RHYTHM STICK CHALLENGES

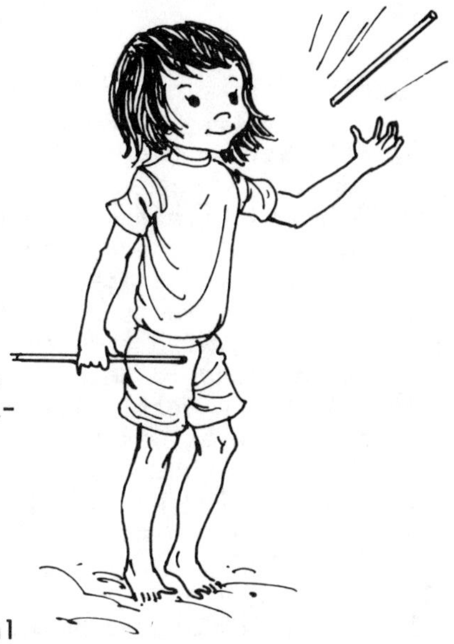

PERFORMANCE OBJECTIVES

By performing the following challenges, student demonstrates abilities of hand-eye coordination, rhythm, laterality, directionality, body image, balance, and finger dexterity.

EQUIPMENT

Classroom set of rhythm sticks.

GENERAL INFORMATION

Rhythm Sticks can provide a valuable addition to any physical education program regardless of the grade level you are working at. The sticks are often referred to as "Lummi Sticks" which is a rhythm game played by moving sticks through various patterns in time to a chant. The "Lummi Sticks" rhythm game, however, is just one of the countless ways of using the sticks to improve the physical coordination of students. Rhythm Sticks can be used to provide students with a wide range of challenges starting with simple basic tasks and progressing to activities requiring increasing amounts of dexterity and coordination.

PROCEDURE

1) May use a circle formation or scatter formation.
2) Students may be seated, kneeling, or standing depending on the types of activities planned.
3) Start by having each student work with only one stick and then progress to 2 sticks per student.
4) Students should work individually at first, but gradually introduce partner activities and then small group experiences.
5) Involvement of all the students in the lesson is the key to success! Enough sticks should be available for each student to have one or 2 depending on the tasks presented.

ONE STICK CHALLENGES

FINE-MOTOR FINGER DEXTERITY

1) Move stick around in a circular motion using fingers. Now move stick in opposite direction. Exchange hands and perform the same tasks. (Try it holding stick vertically and then horizontally.)
2) Finger crawling up and down the tree. Hold stick vertically and move fingers up and down the stick. (Exchange hands and perform the same task.)
3) Twirl like a baton in front of body, to the side, and above. Exchange hands and perform the same tasks.
4) Spin stick on floor. Try both directions. (Perform task using the other hand.)

HAND-EYE REACTION

1) Toss from hand to hand. (Try to track stick with eyes without moving head.)
2) Lift stick up, release above head and catch above head using same hand. (Perform same task using other hand.)

3) Flip stick in air turning it over one time only and catch using the same hand. Use an easy toss. (Perform same task using other hand.)
4) Flip stick in air turning it over 2 times and catch using same hand. (Try using other hand.)
5) Hold stick in front of body at eye level (horizontally) with one hand at each end. Release and catch with one hand before it hits the floor. (Alternate hands when attempting to catch stick.)
6) Hold stick in front of body at eye level (horizontally) using just one hand. Release and catch with the same hand before stick hits the floor. To make it more challenging, student should attempt to catch it below waist level. (Try using other hand.)
7) Hold stick vertically in one hand with arm held straight above head. Release stick and reach across body with opposite hand and attempt to catch before it hits the floor. (Reverse hands and try the same task.)
8) From sitting position, hold stick vertically, bounce on floor and catch. (Perform task using other hand.)

AGILITY
1) Pass stick around body exchanging hands. Quickly change directions on given signal.
2) Pass stick around the knees exchanging hands. Quickly change directions on given signal.
3) Pass stick in and out legs in a figure-eight pattern. Quickly change directions on a given signal.
4) Hold stick horizontally in front of body with one hand at each end. Quickly step over stick with each foot without releasing ends, and then reverse procedure by stepping back again to starting position.

BALANCE
1) Balance stick horizontally on 4 fingers, then 3 fingers, 2 fingers, and one finger. Try the opposite hand.
2) Balance stick on other body parts. Start at top of head, then go to forehead, nose, chin, shoulder, knee, foot.
3) Balance stick vertically on palm, then on fingers. (Try other hand.)
4) Balance stick on various body parts and walk forward, backward, sideways, etc.

STICK TAPPING
1) Leader taps out a sound pattern and students attempt to repeat same pattern. (Good auditory training.)
2) Student holds stick, taps end on floor and flips in air one turn and catches stick using same hand. (Try using other hand.) Progress to 2 taps and a flip, etc.
3) Student holds stick, taps end on floor, flips stick in the air, catches it and taps bottom end of stick on the floor. (Try other hand.) Progress to 2 taps, etc.
4) Alternate hands performing Challenge #2 and #3 above using an easy toss when exchanging hands. Try to keep up a definite rhythmic beat.

STICK AND BALL
Pair off students and have them seated facing each other with legs extended and apart. Each set of partners should have one ball (tennis ball, rubber ball, etc.) to use.
1) Students attempt to hit ball back and forth along the floor. They start fairly close to each other.
2) Students move further away from each other as skill is obtained.
3) Each student sets up one stick as a target. Each partner attempts to hit ball with other stick and knock over partner's stick.
4) In standing position each student attempts to hit ball with stick and keep it bouncing. This is a more advanced skill task.

TWO STICK CHALLENGES

FINE-MOTOR FINGER DEXTERITY

Perform same tasks as listed for activities using only one stick, but have one rhythm stick in each hand. Both hands are now active at the same time which promotes bilaterality.

HAND-EYE REACTION

Perform same tasks as listed for activities using only one stick, except for Challenge #5, but have one rhythm stick in each hand. Both hands are now active at the same time (bilateral movements). In addition to these tasks the following challenges are fun to try.

1) Hammer and nail. Hold one stick which is the hammer and the other stick which represents the nail. Use the hammer to hit the nail down through the hole formed by cupping the hand. (Try hammering with the opposite hand.)
2) Perform the hammer and nail task with the eyes closed. (Tactile and kinesthetic senses now play a primary role.)
3) Hold both sticks in front of body horizontally and hit ends together. Try alternating ends of the sticks when hitting them together. (Palms down, palms up, etc.)
4) Perform Challenge #3 above with the eyes closed.

AGILITY

Set both sticks on the floor in front of body and take a kneeling position.

1) Pick one stick up and begin passing it around your body. Set it down in front of body and do same movement with the other stick. See how fast you can perform the task. Quickly change directions on a given signal.
2) Perform Challenge #1 above with the eyes closed.

BALANCE

1) Balance one stick on each shoulder and walk in various patterns. Try other body parts such as back of hands, wrists, ears, etc.
2) Balance both sticks on the floor at the same time. Walk figure-eight pattern around and between sticks without knocking them over.
3) Make a "T" by balancing one stick on the floor, and placing other stick in balance position on top of it. Now remove top stick of "T" without knocking down the bottom stick.
4) Hold one stick vertically in hand and attempt to balance other stick on top of it. (Sticks are placed end to end.)

STICK TAPPING

1) Leader taps out a sound pattern using both sticks at the same time or alternating sticks. Students attempt to repeat same pattern.
2) Students tap sticks on the floor (front), then click together. Pattern repeats continually with regular rhythmic beat.
3) Students tap sticks on the floor (front), then click together, then flip over and catch sticks. Repetition of pattern continues in rhythmic beat.
4) Students tap sticks on the floor (front), click together, flip over and catch, followed by tapping bottom ends of sticks down on the floor. Cues are front, together, flip, down. Repetition of pattern continues in rhythmic beat.
5) Add side tap to pattern in Challenge #4 above. This is the same as a front tap except that arms go out to sides. Cues are front, together, flip, down, side.
6) Add cross tap to pattern in Challenge #5 above. Forearms cross in front of body, tap sticks to floor.

This collection of Rhythm Stick Challenges is not intended as an exhaustive listing of stick activities. Obviously as you work and experiment with the rhythm sticks, new ideas will present themselves. The students themselves when allowed to explore, will quickly discover and create other movement tasks.

PARACHUTE CHALLENGES

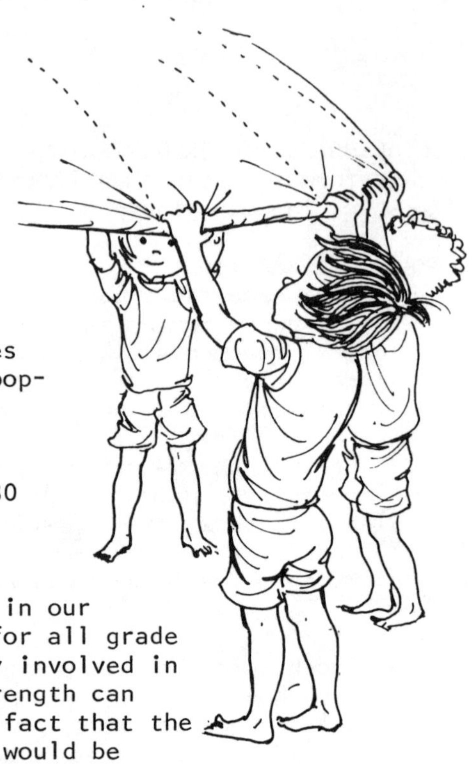

PERFORMANCE OBJECTIVES

By performing the following challenges, student demonstrates arm and shoulder strength, flexibility, group spirit and cooperation, and basic locomotor skills.

EQUIPMENT

Parachute and balls. Note that parachute should be 16 to 30 feet in diameter depending on size of class or group.

GENERAL INFORMATION

The parachute represents an exciting catalyst for movement in our physical education programs. It can be used successfully for all grade levels. An entire class can be continuously and vigorously involved in parachute play and all students regardless of skill and strength can participate successfully. Teachers should be aware of the fact that the parachute lends itself to both indoor and outdoor use. It would be difficult to find a more beneficial fun producing activity for rainy day use, if adequate space is available.

The umbrella part of the "chute" which is called the canopy is the only part used. To begin activity, students line up around the canopy and grasp it with both hands at a seam.

SAFETY PRECAUTIONS

1) Participants should be instructed to hold on to the edge of the chute at all times unless instructed to let go.
2) Stress having the participants look where they are going at all times.
3) Never toss a child up and down on the parachute.
4) Do not allow "horseplay" on the part of any student or students. This will ruin the enjoyment for the rest of the class. (Example: carelessly running around under the parachute.)

TEACHING SUGGESTIONS

1) Begin your lesson by having the entire class stand around the edge of the parachute and grip the canopy at the seams.
2) When inflating the chute, have the class hold it at waist level, then squat and seal the edge against the ground or floor surface. The teacher should immediately count "one, 2, stretch", and on the command "stretch" the whole class must rise and extend their arms high above their heads. The teacher may wish to substitute other commands such as "up" in place of "stretch" but the important thing is to get the canopy as high over-head as possible.
3) Stress the fact that the whole class must work together as a team in order to get good results.
4) Use definite commands for inflating, deflating, etc., so that all students respond at the same instance.

GROUP STUNT CHALLENGES

The most exciting parachute activities involve a cooperative group effort in which the canopy is inflated with air. The billowing chute is an emotionally satisfying experience for all participants.

BASIC INFLATION

Hands are at waist level holding canopy. On signal to begin, students squat and seal chute on ground. On command "one-2-stretch", the arms are thrust overhead. The object is to get as much air as possible under the canopy. When the center of the canopy comes down and touches the floor, repeat the stunt trying to get an even better inflation. This stunt is the basic pattern for other stunts listed.

BALLOONING

The students inflate the chute as in "Basic Inflation" and then walk forward 3 steps toward the center. (Teacher may wish to cue the students by saying, "In! 1-2-3!". Students hold on to the parachute and as it starts to descend, the teacher can give the command "Out! 1-2-3!".

MUSHROOM

The idea of this group stunt is to inflate the parachute and then quickly pull the edges down to the floor (or ground) sealing off the rapid escape of air. The class should continue to hold the edges down tight until the center of the canopy descends to the floor. You may wish to have a contest between 2 teams to see which one can keep the mushroom inflated the longest. The name "Mushroom" comes from the shape of the canopy when sealed with air inside. Have the class try it from both a stationary position and walking 3 steps in before sealing it.

IGLOO

In this stunt, the participants seal themselves inside of the canopy. The parachute is inflated and the students walk 3 steps forward. They quickly turn and re-grasp the chute on the inside edge and then kneel down holding the edge against the ground. The students remain sealed inside the chute until it begins to descend, whereupon they stand holding the chute and duck under to the outside. You may wish to try numbering the students by 2's with one group sealing themselves inside and one group sealing themselves outside.

SUNFLOWER

The parachute is inflated and the students take 3 steps forward. They quickly bring the parachute down and kneel on the outside edge. (The chute should be sealed in the shape of a mushroom.) All students should now join hands and on the commands "In" and "Out", they lean forward and back to represent a sunflower opening and closing.

FLY AWAY

The parachute is inflated and the participants take one step forward. On the command, "Release!", they let go of the canopy which should remain suspended in air for a few seconds before floating to the ground.

GHOST CITY

This stunt is actually a continuation of "Fly Away". Students are instructed not to run after the parachute after it is released, but instead they hold their positions to find out whether there are any ghosts in the class. This occurs when the parachute descends down over the heads of one or more students creating a ghost effect.

CONDITIONING CHALLENGES

Perhaps the most beneficial use of the parachute is in developing physical fitness and this is especially true in terms of improving strength and flexibility of the arm and shoulder girdle muscles in isometric and isotonic conditioning activities. Below are listed some of the most popular exercises performed with the parachute.

BICEP BUILDER

With one leg forward, students plant their feet firmly and lean back, using palms up grip, with arms almost fully extended. On a signal to begin, students pull the chute towards themselves without moving their feet or jerking the chute. The pulling should continue as hard as possible for 6 seconds. Teacher should count aloud and offer encouragement for holding it. Use palms down grip for variation.

WILD HORSE PULL

Students turn with back to the chute and grasp the edge of the canopy with a palms down grip. With one foot forward and one back, they plant their feet firmly on the ground and lean forward. On a signal (whistle) they should pull as hard as they can. You may wish to make team competition out of this exercise by seeing if one half of the parachute can pull the other half in their direction.

OCEAN WAVES

Participants hold the parachute at waist level and, on a signal, slowly begin shaking the chute up and down. The tempo should gradually be increased. Have the participants pull back on the chute as they shake it. A variation for greater arm action is to have the students kneel and then shake it up and down.

SKY HIGH PULL

Participants start with the parachute held at waist level using a palms down grip. They should spread the feet for balance and on signal slowly lift the parachute up until the arms are fully extended overhead. Using just the arms and shoulders (feet, waist, and back do not move) all pull back and hold firmly for 6 seconds. Use the palms up grip for variation.

WRIST ROLL

The parachute is held at waist level (arms extended) with a palms down grip. On a signal to begin, all participants begin slowly rolling the edge of the canopy toward the center. Stress that the group stays together, and at the same time the canopy must be kept tight by pulling a little before each roll of the wrists.

STRAIGHT ARM PULLOVER

Starting position is with the parachute held at waist level using a palms down grip. Feet are shoulder distance apart and on a signal to begin, the arms are extended slowly overhead. Participants should breath in slowly in rhythm with the arm lift. At the point of full extension, the arms are slowly lowered to starting position and participants should exhale. This complete action is repeated at an even tempo for a given number of repetitions.

BEND AND STRETCH

Students hold chute at waist level with palms down grip. On a signal to begin they bend forward touching the edge of the canopy to their toes (count of one). On a count of 2, they extend arms overhead stretching as far as possible. On the count of 3, the students bend forward at the waist and again touch toes. They return to overhead extended arm position on the count of 4. This represents one completed repetition of the exercise.

PUSH-UPS

Students inflate chute and form a mushroom by sealing the edges to the ground. They take push-up position with hands holding the edges tight on the ground. Students perform push-ups by command from the teacher with the chute inflated in the shape of a mushroom.

MODIFIED SQUAT THRUSTS

Performed in the same manner as in "Push-Ups" above except that students extend legs straight back from squat position on the count of one and return to squat position on the count of 2. Count of 3, legs are again extended straight back and on the count of 4 return to squat position. This is one complete 4-count repetition. Students do not come to a standing position as in a regular squat thrust.

TUG-OF-WAR

The parachute is first of all rolled into one long unit similar to a rope. 2 teams are selected, and one team lines up along each half of the parachute. The activity is then conducted as a regular tug-of-war with the students pulling on a given signal to begin. The nylon chute is extremely strong and can be used safely for this activity.

PARACHUTE GAME CHALLENGES

Many of the popular low organized games which are a standard part of our elementary school physical education programs can be readily adapted for use with the parachute. Using the parachute provides a novel approach to presenting games and makes them even more exciting for participants.

POPCORN

3 to 5 rubber balls are placed on the parachute. Students shake the parachute up and down attempting to pop the balls up into the air, but the object is *not* to let them come off the parachute.

BALL SHAKE

The class is divided into 2 equal teams with one team gripping each half of the canopy at the edges. A number of light balls are placed on top of the canopy (rubber balls, tennis balls, beach balls, etc.). On a signal to begin, each team attempts to shake the balls off on the other team's side of the chute. Participants may not use their hands to keep the balls from leaving the canopy. One point is awarded each time a ball leaves the chute and touches the ground.

SURFING (RIDE THE WAVES)

One ball is placed on the edge of the parachute. Students slowly raise and lower the parachute creating a wave effect. The object is to make the ball *roll* around the perimeter of the parachute without losing control. This game requires much teamwork.

NUMBERS EXCHANGE

The students are numbered by 5's or 6's depending on the size of the class. The chute is inflated and as it reaches the maximum height a number is called out. Everyone with that number must leave his/her place on the chute and change places with another student having the same number. All exchanging takes place under the canopy. Students must get to another place before the chute descends and touches their bodies. Penalties may or may not be imposed. Students in lower grades will probably have difficulty getting the chute high enough to run under. For extremeley large groups, it is better to use more numbers so that fewer students are moving about under the parachute. Running, skipping, hopping, jumping, and other locomotor movements can be incorporated into this game.

NUMBERS RACE

The class is divided into 2 equal teams. Each team counts off consecutively. The parachute is inflated and the teacher calls a number. The person on each team whose number is called must travel around the outside of the parachute and return to his place before the center of the chute touches the ground. The teacher should vary the type of locomotor skill used in moving around the chute. Teacher may wish to award one point to the first player returning to his or her own position.

STEAL THE BACON

A bean bag or other small object is placed under the chute at approximately the middle or center of the canopy. The class is divided into 2 equal teams and each player has a team number. The parachute is inflated and at its highest point the teacher calls a number or numbers. Players who have the number called must attempt to secure the bean bag and get back to their position without being tagged by the opponent. Also, if the chute descends on them while under the canopy, no points are awarded. A player who successfully gets back to his/her team position without being tagged or touched by the descending chute, scores one point for his team.

SPECIAL NOTATION

Many other games such as Circle Chase, Dodge Ball, Mouse Trap, and Gray Owl can also be easily adapted to using the parachute.

BASIC LOCOMOTION CHALLENGES

Students in elementary schools, especially the kindergarten and primary grades, need exposure to a variety of challenging and motivating movement experiences. The parachute serving as a catalyst can offer students many fun-filled opportunities for practicing and perfecting basic locomotor skills such as running, hopping, and skipping.

GENERAL APPROACH

Students grasp the edge of the parachute at a seam and use one hand (right or left) designated by the teacher. The teacher has many options in regards to direction that may be used. These options include the following: a) Circle forward in the line of direction; b) Circle backwards; c) Circle forward, on a signal, change griping hands and reverse the line of direction; d) Circle forward and on a signal, move backwards; e) Move in towards the center of the chute and back out; and f) Other combinations using the above listed directions.

LOCOMOTOR SKILLS TO BE STRESSED

a) Walking	b) Running/jogging	c) Hopping	d) Jumping
e) Leaping	f) Skipping	g) Galloping	h) Sliding

OTHER SUGGESTIONS

1) Appropriate music may be played to provide added fun and environment.
2) The chute may be alternately raised and lowered as the students move around in a circle.
3) A merry-go-round can be created by alternating student movements.
4) Simple dances can be developed incorporating basic locomotor skills with the parachute serving as the focal point for movement.

MOVEMENT EXPLORATION CHALLENGES

Movement Exploration refers to a problem solving approach in which the students are challenged to think and then move in many different and creative ways. The teacher asks such leading questions as Who Can? Can You? Show me how! , etc. Listed below are just some of the many possibilities to explore movement.

1) How would you make waves using the parachute?
2) Can you run in a circle holding the chute extended overhead with the right hand?
3) Show me how you would hop around in a circle alternating from your right to your left foot (gripping the chute).
4) Can you grip the chute with both hands palm down and raise and lower the chute with arms extended?
5) How fast can you roll the canopy towards the center with the chute kept tight at all times?
6) Show me how you would raise the chute overhead, then release it, and regrasp it while floating in space.
7) Can you cross your arms and pull back hard on the chute while I count to 6?
8) Show me how you can hold the parachute at a high level while running at a low level.
9) Can you perform sit-ups while grasping the edge of the chute? Who can do 10 sit-ups?
10) Can you inflate the chute and run to your left? (Repeat to the right.)
11) Can you inflate the chute and hop 3 steps in, and then 3 steps back out?
12) Can you show me a new activity using the parachute?

SPECIAL ACTIVITIES

There are many other special types of parachute activities which teachers may wish to experiment with in their physical education program. They are listed below without a detailed description. Letting the imagination take charge will certainly produce many more interesting and meaningful experiences for students.

TUMBLING

Mats are placed under the parachute. Members of the class hold the chute in the inflated position while other pupils perform forward rolls, backward rolls, animal stunts, etc.

PYRAMIDS

Class is divided into teams of 6. Each team tries to build a pyramid under the parachute before it comes down from an inflated position and touches them. Mats are placed under the chute for the students to perform on. Teams must be allowed time to practice their pyramids without the parachute so that each member of the team knows exactly what to do.

SELF-TESTING

Students can be given the challenge of ball bouncing, rope jumping, etc., under the inflated chute.

LONG JUMP ROPE

The parachute can be rolled up in the form of a long jump rope. As a long rope, students can run and jump over it, and then crawl under it coming back. They can also hop and jump back and forth over the chute when it is lying on the ground like an extended rope. Many other movement patterns can be presented using the chute in this manner.

DANCE STEPS

Basic dance steps such as the schottische, step hop, 2 step, polka, and mazurka can be practiced using the parachute as a stimulus for movement. Music will add greatly to this activity.

STILT CHALLENGES

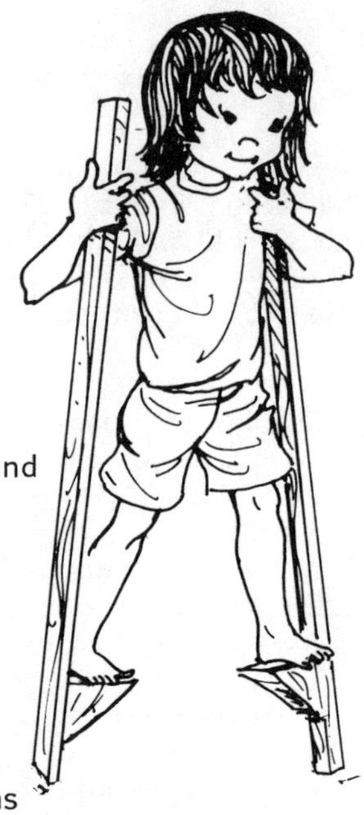

PERFORMANCE OBJECTIVES

By performing the following challenges, student demonstrates static and dynamic balance, agility, strength, and foot-eye coordination.

EQUIPMENT

Classroom set of stilts.

GENERAL INFORMATION

The use of stilts in school physical education programs is becoming more and more prevalent throughout the United States. With greater stress being placed on the development of purposeful movement programs for students of all age levels, the value of stilts in enhancing the self-image and self-confidence of students is gaining wide acceptance. Stilts have especially been singled out for their contribution to balance training, although teachers have discovered stilts can also make significant contributions in the areas of agility, strength, and foot-eye coordination.

Balance training should be a basic and important part of motor development programs. Balance underlies all movement tasks, and is vital to specific sport skills such as throwing and catching. In order for balance to improve significantly, specific training must be introduced into our physical education programs.

Three important factors underlie the use of stilts in promoting balance and motor-fitness:

1) Balance is learned by imbalance. When using stilts, the student is placed in a situation where adjustment in the center of gravity must be made to achieve total balance.
2) Balance is improved by continuously adding to the task difficulty. In using stilts, a constant stress is placed on the student to maintain balance. By adding simple challenges to the stilt program, the task difficulty or challenge is ever present.
3) Balance programs must incorporate activities which are geared to promote both static balance (stationary) and dynamic balance (moving). Stilts can easily be used in a stationary position or in locomotor experiences to challenge balance.

TEACHING SUGGESTIONS

Below are listed some helpful hints for teachers to use when first introducing students to stilts.

1) Have the students line up with their backs against a wall and stilts in hands ready to mount. The wall will serve as a support and reinforcement for the students.
2) Students should place strong leg (dominant leg) on stirrup (foot support) of stilt first and then step up with other leg to catch their balance. They can lean back against a wall, if necessary, to maintain balance.
3) Emphasize that stilts are held in tight against the legs and that body should be kept straight (tall) and fairly rigid (firm) at first.
4) In order to get a "feel" for the stilts, ask the students to shift weight from one stilt to the other stilt. (Sort of rocking back and forth on the stilts.)
5) Once the students begin to feel secure on the stilts, encourage the students to walk a few steps out from the wall.
6) After the students are able to walk a short distance and maintain balance, ask them to mount the stilts without use of the wall and attempt to move in different directions.

7) With a little practice and encouragement from the teacher, the students will soon be moving with ease and confidence on the stilts and excitement will fill the air.

MOVEMENT EXPLORATION CHALLENGES

In movement exploration the student is presented with verbal challenges or problems to be solved. The instructor's tools are leading questions, some of which have many answers. The teacher must give constant encouragement and praise with each student challenged to work within their own capacity level.

1) Can you place both feet on your stilts and hold your balance?
2) Can you keep your balance on both stilts until I count to 3? 5? Etc.
3) Who can take one step forward on your stilts?
4) Show me if you can take several steps before dismounting.
5) I would like to see if anyone can walk backwards on their stilts.
6) This time, see if you can walk backwards a greater distance before dismounting.
7) Who can walk several steps forward and then backward without dismounting?
8) Can anyone here walk sideways on their stilts?
9) Can you walk sideways again and cross your feet over as you move sidewards?
10) On the hardtop can you walk along a painted line? Around a circle? A 4-square court?
11) Can you make yourself very low on your stilts? Now, very tall?
12) At the hopscotch area, who can walk a hopscotch court by placing just one stilt in each of the squares or forms?
13) Can you walk in rhythm to the music? (Marching on stilts.)
14) Show me how quickly you can move from this line to that line. How slowly can you travel this same distance, but remember, you must keep moving forward?
15) Who can walk with their stilts very close together?
16) Who can walk in many different directions on their stilts? Now, each time I blow the whistle, change directions.
17) How would you change speed? Fast to slow, slow to fast, etc.
18) Who can do something different on their stilts?

OBSTACLE COURSE CHALLENGES

Obstacles of different shapes and sizes present a natural motivating challenge to the student on stilts. By increasing the distance to walk around an obstacle course, you are able to incorporate endurance training into the stilt program. Improved spatial orientation is achieved by arranging obstacles which have a limited space or opening for the student to relate to.

1) Set out hoops, ropes, traffic cones, boxes, tires, waste baskets, plastic bottles, etc.
2) Playground equipment such as the tetherball poles, basketball backboard support poles, and apparatus equipment may be incorporated into your obstacle course.
3) Additional motivation for students needing a greater challenge can be achieved by using a stop watch to time them.
4) Occassionally allow the students opportunities to make up their own obstacle course.

CONTEST CHALLENGES

Contests provide an opportunity for students to engage in enjoyable competition. They help to develop self-confidence, agility and the ability to react and think quickly.

CIRCLE BALANCING

Draw several 18 inch circles on the hardtop using chalk. One participant is lined up at each circle. Stirrup end of both stilts are placed in the circle with the performer holding other end of stilts in hands ready to mount on command. Anyone losing balance and forced to get off the stilts, or step out of their circle is eliminated.

STILT ROOSTER FIGHT

Mark off a series of 5 foot circles. Opponents are paired off 2 to a circle. Contestants place end of stilts in circle, opposite from each other and ready to mount. On command, they mount, and by bumping, try to force opponent from the circle or off stilts. The contestant staying on stilts and in the circle is the winner. This has to be carefully supervised!

25 OR 50 YARD RACE

Contestants line up on starting line in a position ready to mount stilts. On signal, they mount stilts and travel to the finish line.

CROOKED LINE RACE

Chalk lines are marked on hard top area. Performer must follow the line with one stilt on each side.

STILT KICK FOR HEIGHT

Contestant must mount stilts and on a given signal attempts to kick one stilt as high as possible without dismounting stilts. The instructor must measure the height of the kick and records this score. Each contestant should be given at least 2 trials.

RELAY CHALLENGES

Relays have built-in motivation for participants and provide an opportunity for all students to practice skills with a limited amount of equipment necessary. Relays help to develop group spirit and add fun and variety to the physical education program.

SHUTTLE

Any number of teams may be used with members of each team divided into 2 groups. Two parallel lines 30 to 50 feet apart are used as restraining lines. One half of the players for each team line up in file formation behind one restraining line and the other half of each team lines up behind the opposite restraining line. Each team needs one pair of stilts. At a signal, the leader for each team mounts his/her stilts and travels across the opposite restraining line. The first player for each team at the opposite line then mounts the stilts and travels back. The relay continues in this manner until all players have returned to their original position. The first team to finish scores one point for their team.

PIN TOPPLE

Players are in relay formation (single file) with each file facing a pin placed 30 to 50 feet away. Each team has one pair of stilts. On a signal to begin, the first player in each file mounts his/her stilts, and travels to the pin opposite his/her file. Players must knock the pin over with one of the stilts and then return to his/her team. The 2nd player in line for each team next mounts the stilts and travels back to the pin. This player must dismount, set up the pin, then mount his/her stilts and return to his/her team. The relay continues in this manner until all players have had their turn. The first file to finish and in a straight line behind their leader, scores one point.

HOOP PATTERN

Use regular relay procedure for organizing teams and place 5 to 7 hoops in a pattern opposite each team. The same pattern should be presented to each team. Examples of patterns are:

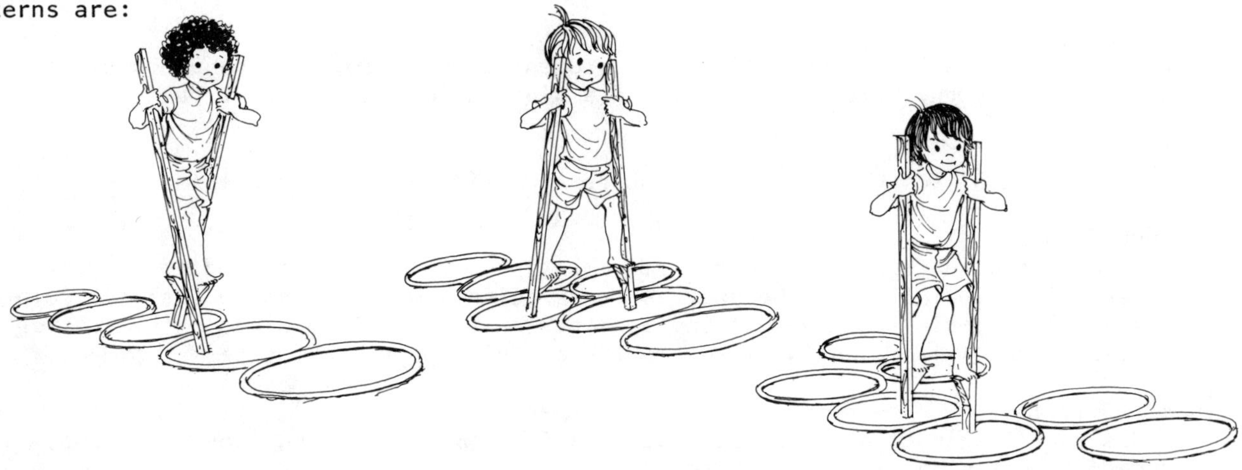

The players on each team in turn must move through the pattern on stilts, keeping the stilts inside of the hoops once they enter the pattern. Teacher may use shuttle formation or regular single file formation.

STILT ROPE STEPPING

Use regular relay procedure for organizing teams and place 4 or 5 individual ropes in parallel formation, opposite each team.

The players on each team must, in turn, walk to the ropes on their stilts and step over the ropes without touching them with their stilts. Each player continues on to a restraining line, turns around without dismounting, and returns to his/her team again stepping over the ropes. If relay is performed in shuttle formation, a player would only pass over the ropes in one direction.

SPECIAL NOTE

The stilt activities listed in this section vary from beginning basic stilt movements to activities requiring a high level of skill. Obviously the degree to which children will be able to participate in the outlined challenges depends on their achieved skill level.

SCARF CHALLENGES

PERFORMANCE OBJECTIVES

By performing the following challenges, student demonstrates eye-hand coordination, creative rhythmic expression, and a wide variety of movement patterns.

EQUIPMENT

Classroom set of scarves 18" to 24" square in a wide variety of colors.

INTRODUCTION

The scarf is a fun and "easy to use" movement prop which can be used to motivate children. Successful manipulation of the scarves comes quickly which leads to positive reinforcement in a highly stimulating movement environment. A wide variety of colorful scarves add to the visual qualities. Adding music to the activity provides further enjoyment.

SCARF ACTIVITIES

1) Use your imagination---what can your scarf become? Floating leaves, clouds, magic carpet, ocean waves, flying kite, etc.
2) Use your imagination---what can *you* become using your scarf? Bull Fighter, Magician, Juggler, Flamingo Dancer, Clown, etc.
3) Can you "draw" in space using your scarf? Try making circles and other shapes, numbers, letters, zig-zag lines, etc.
4) Who can perform exercise movements using their scarf as a prop? Stretching exercises, jumping exercises, twisting exercises, etc.
5) Use your imagination and create beautiful art designs and pictures using your scarf. Lift the scarf up high, release, and let it fall to the ground. Now study the design created, and share with your friends. Is it a fish, a mountain range, sail boat, etc?
6) What types of "tricks" or stunts can you do with your scarf?
7) Explore levels with your scarf. Can you make it move very high in space, very low, between high and low, etc?
8) Try moving about our space (room, auditorium, etc.) using different types of locomotor skills and keep your scarf moving. Running, skipping, jumping, hopping, etc.
9) Pretend you are a juggler and show me how you can lift your scarf up high, release it, and catch it in various ways.
   a) Lift, release, and catch with your preferred hand.
   b) Use your other (less preferred) hand.
   c) Release with one hand and catch with the other.
   d) Release, clap hands, and catch scarf. (Clap once, twice, three times, etc.).
   e) How low to the ground can you catch your scarf?
   f) Who can lift, release the scarf, then touch the body part I call out before catching your scarf? Shoulders, elbows, knees, toes, etc.
   g) Try lifting and releasing scarf, and then turn completely around and catch it.
   h) Tie a knot in one end of your scarf and try some of these challenges. NOTE: Scarf will now be weighted and move faster while falling.
10) Show me how you can catch your scarf on different body parts. Head, elbow, wrist, knee, foot, etc.
11) How quickly can you pass your scarf from hand to hand? Around your waist, around your knees, figure eight between and around knees, etc.
12) Who can keep their scarf floating in space by blowing on it?
13) Mirror Image---I am going to make slow flowing movements with my scarf. Can you follow or copy my movements as if looking into a mirror? NOTE: In mirror image activities follower(s) use opposite hand from leader as if looking into a mirror.
14) Partner Mirror Image---with a partner I would like you to play the mirror image game. One person will lead and the other follows. When I say "Change", switch roles.
15) If adequate numbers of scarves are available, have children explore two scarf and three scarf juggling routines.

TIRE CHALLENGES

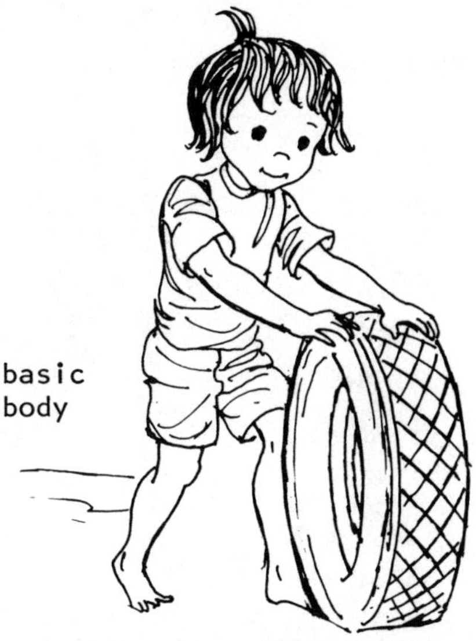

PERFORMANCE OBJECTIVES

By performing the following challenges, student demonstrates basic locomotor skills, motor planning ability, spatial awareness, body image, balance, laterality, directionality, and hand-eye and foot-eye coordination.

EQUIPMENT

Classroom set of bicycle tires.

GENERAL INFORMATION

Tires are among the most versatile, inexpensive, indestructible, and easily obtained teacher tools available for use in the physical education program. They can be used either indoors or out and offer the teacher a means of challenging students in an endless variety of movement tasks. These tasks may be simplified to offer successful participation for the motor deficient student, or designed to challenge the physically gifted. Bicycle tires, due to factors of safety, lightness in handling, and storage, are generally considered to be more practical than car tires, but certainly both types of tires have their own unique qualities which make them more desirable for specific types of experiences.

TEACHING SUGGESTIONS

1) There are many approaches to using tires, but probably the most effective way is to use them as a part of various movement stations or circuits.
2) Tires are very easy to incorporate into an obstacle course and may be used in many different positions to provide exciting challenges.
3) If enough tires are available so that each student has his/her own individual tire, then the teacher may wish to use a movement exploration approach using verbal challenges such as "Who can?", "Show me how...", etc., as recommended in the introduction to this book.
4) Tire relays, games, and contests are extremely popular with students and offer variety to the physical education program.
5) If possible, it is best to spray paint the tires various colors to add visual cues to the challenges. Color in itself is an effective motivator of movement. Many types of perceptual-motor learning can be structured into the program using colors as meaningful symbols.
6) Acquiring various sizes of tires adds space relationships to the challenges offered to students.

MOVEMENT PATTERN CHALLENGES

Tires are placed in patterns and students are challenged to move through the patterns using various forms of locomotion. Examples of patterns which might be used are shown on the next page. Jump standards or cross bars may be added to the tire patterns to enhance skill and make the challenge more complex.

Pattern 1 | Pattern 2 | Pattern 3 | Pattern 4 | Pattern 5 | Pattern 6

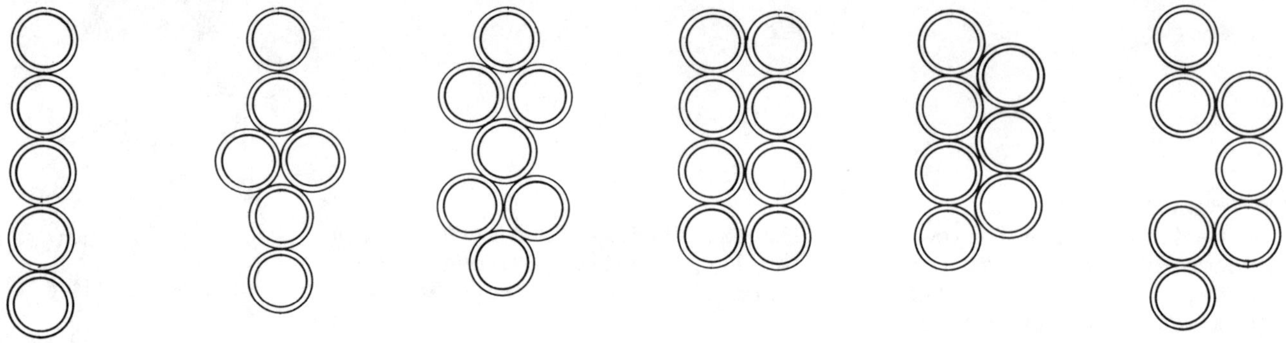

1) Step in and out of the tires moving from one to another without touching the sides of the tires.
2) Run through the tires placing one foot in each tire. Can you run on top of the edges of the tires?
3) Jump in an out of the tires with your feet together. Can you jump forward? Backward? Sideways? Etc.
4) Hop in and out of the tires using the right foot. Also try the left foot.
5) Creep through the tires on your hands and knees placing hands and knees in tire openings. Can you creep on top of the tires?
6) Move through the tire patterns imitating the movements of various animals.
   a) Dog Run on hands and feet.
   b) Bear Walk on hands and feet.
   c) Rabbit Hop moving hands and then feet.
   d) Frog Jump pushing off from toes and landing on toes.
   e) Crab Walk with stomach up placing hands and feet in tire opening.
7) Place tires at various distances apart.
   a) Broad jump (long jump) from tire to tire.
   b) Run and leap from tire to tire.
8) Variations of the previous challenges.
   a) Points of contact or body parts. Can you move through the tires using 3 points of contact? Can you use 4 body parts?
   b) Find a different way of moving through the tires.
   c) Walk through the tires placing the right foot in tires on the right side and the left foot in the tires on the left side and verbalize right or left as each foot lands in the tire opening.
   d) Perform half-turns (twisting jumps) while moving in and out of tire openings.

TARGET CHALLENGES

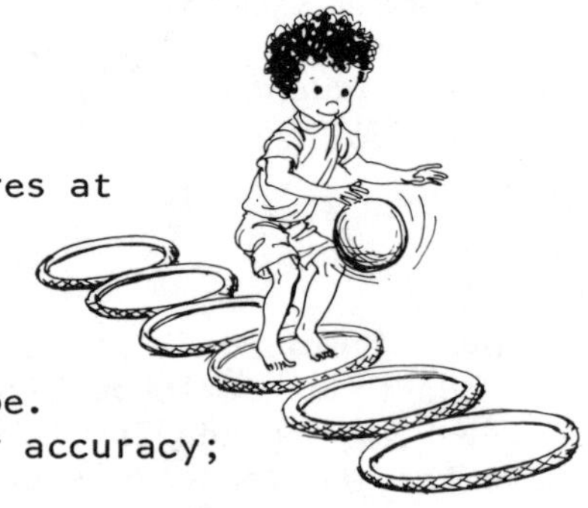

1) Toss bean bags into tires placed flat on the floor. Place tires at different distances. Try matching colors, toss red bean bag into red tire, etc.
2) Bounce and catch rubber ball in tires placed end to end.
3) Dribble ball in tires placed end to end.
4) Throw or pitch balls through tire suspended (hanging) by a rope. Examples: football passing for accuracy; softball pitching for accuracy; tennis ball overhand throw for accuracy; etc.
5) Roll tires and have partners attempting to throw ball through a moving target.
6) Kick balls for accuracy through tires of various sizes.

CONTEST CHALLENGES

1) Tire rolling for accuracy using a circle on the playground. Object: To make tire stop within the circle.
2) Tire rolling for distance.
3) Tire accuracy roll between 2 parallel lines.
4) Tire bowling attempting to knock over bowling pins placed in triangle formation.
5) Tire speed rolling using hands to roll tire between 2 goal lines. Try using stop watch for time.
6) Tire agility crawling. Object: To see how fast you can move through 3 or 4 tires of various sizes.
7) Tire Leap Frog. Object: To straddle-jump over a rolling tire without touching the tire.

COMBATIVE CHALLENGES

TIRE WRESTLING

2 or 4 tires are placed on the grass or mats so that they are touching. One student stands in each tire and on a signal they attempt to push or pull each other so that at least one part of the body touches the ground or mat outside the tire.

TIRE PULL

2 opponents grab hold of the tire and attempt to pull each other across a restraining line.

TIRE CREEP

2 opponents are on their hands and knees facing in opposite directions with a tire over one of their feet and legs. They attempt to creep forward on a signal and pull each other over a restraining line.

TIRE BUMPING

2 to 4 students each place a bicycle tire over their heads and shoulders and on a signal attempt to hop forward on one foot only. Arms are across chest and, holding tire with each hand, they attempt to bump each other and knock their opponent (or opponents) off balance so that both feet touch the ground. (Use on grass or mats for safety.)

RELAY CHALLENGES

TIRE ROLLING

Roll tires using left hand down and right hand back.

TIRE CARRY

Partners carry tire with each partner holding one side.

TIRE SHUTTLE

Each runner carries a bike tire and hands it off to the next runner.

TIRE SCRAMBLE

Each team member must run to a bike tire, pull it down over his/her head, step out and run to tag the next player in line.

TIRE ROBOT

Each team member must run with tire around the waist down to a goal line and back.

TIRE AND BALL

A tire with ball resting within opening is placed on the center line which is located between 2 restraining lines. (Each team has a tire and ball.) Each team member must run down to tire, pick up the ball, dribble it across the opposite restraining line, then run back , place ball within the tire, and finally tag the hand of the next runner.

MOVEMENT EXPLORATION CHALLENGES

Each student must have a bicycle tire to work with. This same approach can be used with hoops.

1) How fast can you run around your tire?
2) Can you balance on one foot within your tire? Now try the opposite foot. Close your eyes and see how long you can hold your balance.
3) Can you jump up and down within your tire and go higher with each jump?
4) Who can hop on one foot within their tire? Try the opposite foot. Can you hop 5 times on your right foot, then 5 times on your left foot?
5) Show me how you can jump out and back in your tire moving in different directions. (Forward, backward, sideways in various combinations.)
6) How would you do a straddle jump with feet moving outside the tire and then back together inside the tire?
7) Walk around the rim (or top edge) of the tire maintaining good balance. Can you move backwards?
8) Run and jump into your tire landing in a crouch position.
9) From a crouch position inside your tire, see how far out of your tire you can travel using a frog jump.
10) How far can you broad jump (long jump) out of your tire? Now turn and face your tire. Can you long jump back to the center of your tire?
11) On a signal, hop out of your tire and continue to hop around your tire on the same foot. On the next signal, quickly change directions and change the foot you are hopping on.
12) Place your hands on the floor inside of your tire and walk around the outside.
13) Who can use one hand for a pivot (or balance point) inside of tire and move feet around the outside of the tire? Can you change hands and change direction of movement?
14) With your back to the ground and stomach toward the ceiling, can you move around your tire keeping your feet inside the tire and hands outside? (Crab position.)
15) How small can you make yourself inside the tire? How large? How tall? Etc.
16) Find a way of balancing with 3 body parts touching inside the tire and 2 body parts touching outside the tire. (Use various other combinations.)
17) Can you build a long narrow bridge across your tire using your body? Make a wide bridge, high bridge, a draw bridge, etc.
18) Try a 1/2 body spin inside your tire. Who can make a full spin or turn inside of his/her tire?
19) Working with a partner, can you roll one tire back and forth? Can you coordinate 2 tires?
20) Working with a partner, can you toss and catch a bicycle tire back and forth? Can you coordinate 2 tires using a toss and a catch?

MISCELLANEOUS CHALLENGES

Tires can be used in combination with other pieces of equipment to create purposeful and fun movement experiences. Below are listed some of the many possibilities.

1) Use in combination with incline board and jump box for spatial target to jump into when placed on the floor (mat). Several tires may be used to offer a more difficult challenge.

2) Use with walking boards for stepping in and out of while maneuvering the length of the board.
3) Use in combination with the walking board to bounce a rubber ball into when placed in various positions on the floor alongside of the board. Student must maintain balance, and bounce and catch the ball in each tire while maneuvering the length of the board.
4) Use in conjunction with an inner tube having a canvas cover or a large inner tube as a target to jump into and land with full body control.
5) Use with cross bars or jump standards to offer various types of jumping and hopping challenges.

HELPFUL HINTS

Used and discarded tires can be easily obtained at no cost from local gas stations and bicycle repair stores. Also, students are usually willing to bring old tires to school when asked to contribute.

Although the Tire Challenges in this section cover a wide range of movement experiences using tires, it is not intended to be a complete source of activities. It is hoped that teachers will become acquainted with many interesting and exciting possibilities for using tires in the physical education programs and, in the process, modify or create activities to fit individual needs. Tire games have not been included in this section due to the inumerable possibilities, but certainly, they can become another enjoyable dimension to the use of bicycle tires.

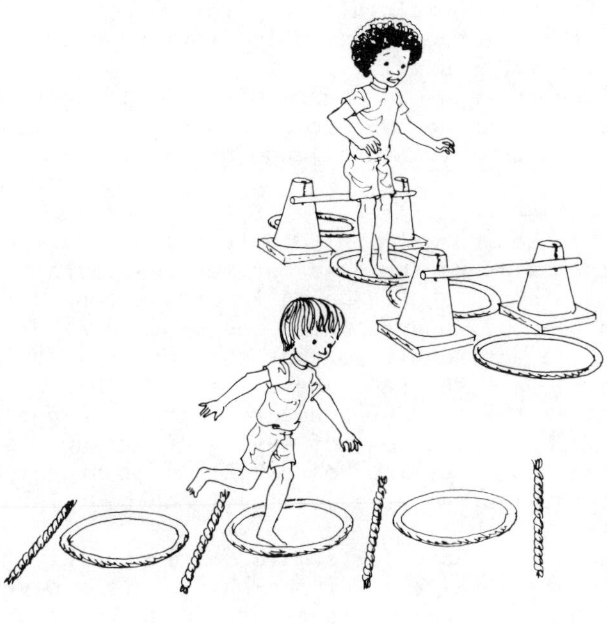

WALKING BOARD CHALLENGES

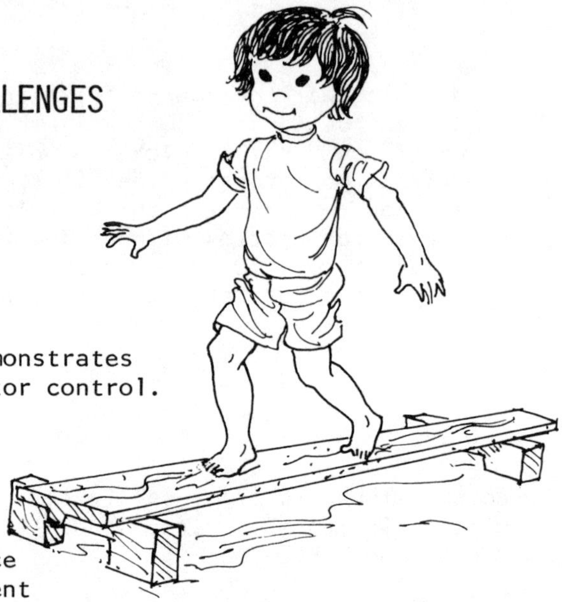

PERFORMANCE OBJECTIVES

By performing the following challenges, student demonstrates balance, laterality, body awareness, and visual-motor control.

EQUIPMENT

Set of low, intermediate, and high walking boards.

GENERAL INFORMATION

The walking board commonly referred to as a "balance beam" is probably the most popular piece of equipment for improving a student's balance. When used by a perceptive teacher, it can become a valuable tool not only for stimulating the balance mechanisms, but also for fostering improved visual motor skills and laterality. Basic principles which should be kept in mind when attempting to improve the balance of students are listed below.

1) Balance is learned by imbalance. The student must be placed in a situation where he or she adjusts his or her center of gravity to achieve total balance.
2) Balance is improved by continuously adding to the task difficulty. Having a student repetitiously walk a balance board where there is no stress or imbalance created is wasting valuable instruction time.
3) Balance tasks are made progressively more difficult by changing the width, height, or angle of the walking surface, using obstacles which require body adjustments, imposing variations in the manner which the eyes are used, requiring changes in the center of gravity, and by requiring the student to use fewer or additional body supports as he or she attempts to maintain equilibrium.
4) Both static (stationary) balance and dynamic (moving) balance should be promoted within the structure of the tasks used.
5) Balance factors include the sensory organs of vision, touch, kinesthesis, and vestibular functioning. The teacher should be aware of the amount of sensory input which must be processed within any given challenge or task.

TEACHING SUGGESTIONS

1) The walking boards should be approximately 10 feet long and constructed so that either a 4 inch side or a 2 inch side can be used for various tasks.
2) The height of the walking board should be an important consideration in planning appropriate challenges. In general, boards which can be used at different heights (preferrably 3 or more heights) are desireable so that changes in visual cues and perception of space can be incorporated into the sequence of tasks. This also helps to promote greater self-confidence as the student conquers fear of height.
3) The walking board should be used as one of several learning stations within a perceptual-motor lesson. By setting up 2 walking boards at different heights, more involvement will take place, and tasks learned at a low level can be reinforced at a higher level in space.
4) In general, most students will be able to move fairly rapidly from the low level (7 inch height) to the intermediate level (11 inch height). After developing confidence and emotional security at the intermediate level, the high board challenge (20 inch height) is eagerly accepted.
5) Some students will require physical contact (holding hand, etc.) when first attempting to maneuver on the board, but gradually remove this "crutch" so the initial fear is overcome.

6) Insist that students walk the board in their bare feet. *No* shoes or socks! This allows for increased tactile and kinesthetic stimulation. Shoes "mask out" sensory information and socks are extremely slippery.
7) The use of obstacles such as bean bags, ropes, bicycle tires, and traffic cones with adjustable cross tubes (cross bars) can provide continuous new challenge and motivation in maneuvering on the board.
8) In general, one student at a time should be on the walking board and movement takes place going in one direction only. Some tasks will require the student to move to one end of the board and back to the starting position, but these tasks are noted within the listed sequence.

SKILLS TO STRESS

1) Student should walk the board slowly so that maximum opportunity for making adjustments in center of gravity is provided. Walking the board fast minimizes the number of times the student must come from imbalance to total balance.
2) Encourage student to keep the chin up so that he or she is *not* watching the feet while walking the board.
3) Eyes should focus on an object at the end of the board so that the eyes are guiding total body movement towards a point of focus. The instructor's hand held at eye level and occassionally shifted slowly sideways or up and down, makes an excellent visual target.
4) When obstacles such as bicycle tires are added to the challenge, the eyes should focus on each obstacle in sequence and shift focal points as the board is maneuvered on.
5) The student should walk the board in bare feet keeping each foot straight on the board with no overhang.
6) When walking backwards, the student feels for the board with the toes of the feet and then allows the heel to come down in contact with the board.
7) When walking sideways, the weight is balanced on the "balls" of the feet.
8) It is important to emphasize good posture with head erect and shoulders back as the student walks the board.
9) The arms should be carried low and slightly out to the side for making easy adjustments in the center of gravity. Comfort is important here! Many students carry their arms extended out sideways at shoulder height, and this tends to tighten up the upper body area and makes it more difficult to maintain balance.
10) When picking up objects such as bean bags or changing levels of body positioning, the student should not stoop over, but rather lowers the hips down keeping the shoulders back.

CHALLENGES

1) Walk forward slowly with eyes focusing on visual target (teacher's hand).
2) Walk forward slowly with hands placed on hips.
3) Walk forward stepping in and out of 2 bicycle tires placed on the walking board. (Use small bicycle tires 18 inches in diameter spaced approximately 4 feet apart.)
4) Walk forward, balance on one foot (stork balance) at center of board, and then continue walking to the end of the board.
5) Walk forward, balance on the left foot in the first bicycle tire, continue walking to the 2nd bicycle tire, balance on the right foot, and walk to the end of the board.
6) Walk forward, step over cross bar placed across center of walking board. (Use traffic cones with adjustable cross tube for obstacles.)
7) Walk forward stepping in and out of first tire, over cross bar, and then in and out of 2nd tire.
8) Walk forward carrying a balance pole (broom handle, etc.) using an overhand grip with hands placed slightly wider than shoulder distance apart. Hold pole at shoulder level.
9) Walk forward carrying a balance pole with weighted object (bucket, clorox bottle, etc.) attached to one end of pole so that the student must make adjustments.
10) Walk forward and step over 4 bean bags spaced evenly along the walking board without looking down at feet. (Bean bags are spaced approximately 2 feet apart along the length of the walking surface.)

11) Walk forward using "snake" rope as visual target. (Student attempts to step into spaces provided by rope without waking up the sleeping snake. Rope is coiled around walking board.)
12) Walk sideways leading with the right foot to the end of the board. On the next turn, walk sideways with the left foot leading. Do *not* cross the feet!
13) Walk sideways to the center of the board with the left foot leading, make a half turn, and walk sideways to the end of the board with the right foot leading.
14) Walk forward to the end of the board with arms out to the sides of the body balancing a bean bag on top of each hand.
15) Walk forward performing a heel-toe balance walk while supporting a bean bag on top of the head.
16) Walk forward to the center of the board, lower the body down and pick up a bean bag, place it on the head and walk to the end of the board.
17) Walk forward, pick up the bean bag and place on the head, then continue walking forward, step over the cross bar, and walk to the end of the board.
18) Walk slowly backwards to the end of the board with the head erect. Student stops when he or she "feels" the end of the board is there.
19) Walk forward to the center of the board, make a half turn and walk backwards to the end of the board.
20) Walk backwards to the end of the board while balancing a bean bag on top of each hand.
21) Walk forward 1/3rd of the way, turn and walk sideways 1/3rd of the way, then turn and walk backwards to the end of the board.
22) Walk forward balancing bicycle tire on each wrist, make a half turn at the center of the board, and walk backward to the end of the board.
23) Walk backwards, step over the first bean bag, make a complete (full) turn at the center of the board, continue to walk backwards stepping over the 2nd bean bag, and walk to the end of the board.
24) Walk forward up to the end of the inclined board, make a half turn and walk forward back down to the starting position. (Remove one support to make board into an inclined walking surface.)
25) Walk backward up to the end of the inclined board, make a half turn and walk backward down to the starting position.
26) Walk forward, step over the first cross bar, continue walking forward and duck under the 2nd cross bar placed at shoulder height and walk to the end of the board.
27) Walk forward, step over the cross bar, make a full turn at the center of the board, continue forward and go through a hoop, and walk to the end of the board.
28) Walk forward carrying a rubber ball held out in front of the body at chest level. (A 7 inch diameter rubber ball is recommended for ball activities on the walking board.)
29) Walk forward to the center of the board carrying a rubber ball, bounce the ball on the floor and catch, continue walking to the end of the board.
30) Walk forward carrying a rubber ball, bounce and catch the ball after every 2 steps. (Ball is bounced on the floor, and not on the walking board.)
31) Walk forward carrying a rubber ball, step over the first cross bar, walk to the center of the board, bounce and catch the ball in tires placed on each side of the board (left side, then right side), walk forward and step over 2nd cross bar, and continue walking to the end of the board.
32) Walk forward carrying a rubber ball, bounce and catch the ball in 4 tires placed on alternate sides of the board. (Left side, right side, left side, and right side.) Have student verbalize correct directions: left side, right side, etc. Tires are spaced evenly alongside the length of the board.

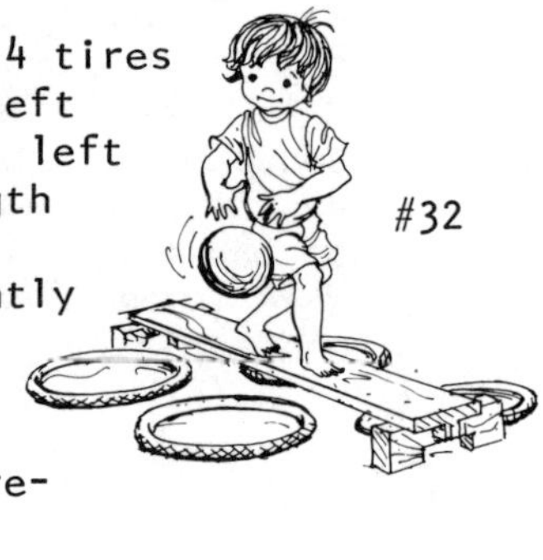

#32

33) Walk slowly forward while tossing and catching a rubber ball slightly above head level. Ball is tossed up after every 2 or 3 steps. (For additional challenge, add hand clapping.)
34) Walk forward carrying a rubber ball, toss and catch with the instructor. (Approximately 3 underhand tosses and catches will be required to navigate the length of the board.)

35) Walk forward carrying a rubber ball, dribble ball 5 times in a hoop placed on the left side of the board, continue walking forward and dribble the ball 5 times in the hoop placed on the right side of the board.
36) Walk forward and dribble the ball continuously on the floor until reaching the end of the board.
37) Walk forward with the eyes tracing a swinging ball moving at eye level at the opposite end of the board. (Use a styrofoam or plastic ball suspended by a cord.) Instructor or aide swings ball slowly from side to side. Stress smooth eye movements from side to side without the head moving!
38) Walk forward to the center of the board, kneel on one knee, rise and walk to the end of the board. (Student should alternate knee action: first turn left knee, 2nd turn right knee, etc.)
39) Walk forward, touch left knee to first bean bag placed on the board, continue walking forward and touch right knee to the 2nd bean bag placed on the board. (Bean bags are spaced approximately 4 feet apart on the walking board.)
40) Walk forward, perform a swan balance on the left foot in the first tire, continue walking to the 2nd tire and perform a swan balance on the right foot. (On the swan balance, student bends forward from the waist and extends arms out sideways with the body supported on one leg only.)
41) Walk forward to the center of the board, balance on one foot for 5 seconds, turn on this same foot and walk backwards to the end of the board.
42) Walk forward balancing on hands and feet until reaching the end of the board. (This is commonly referred to as a "cat walk".)
43) Walk forward while tossing a bean bag from hand to hand like a juggler. Challenge the student to follow bean bag with the eyes and not to move the head.
44) Hop the length of the board moving on the left foot only.
45) Hop the length of the board moving on the right foot only.
46) Walk the length of the board keeping the eyes closed or covered. Instructor or aide should walk alongside of the board to offer assistance, if needed. (If the student is successful with this challenge, offer variations moving sideways and backwards.)
47) Partners join hands with one person walking backwards and the other person walking forwards and walk to the end of the board. When the person walking backwards reaches the end of the board, they return to the starting position, but now they are reversing direction of body movements.
48) Partners start at opposite ends of the board, walk slowly forward to the center of the board, pass each other and continue walking to the end of the board.
49) Partners start walking slowly forward on 2 separate walking boards placed parallel to each other about 4 feet apart. They toss a rubber ball back and forth while walking towards the end of their respective boards.
50) Partners start at opposite ends of 2 separate walking boards and walk towards each other on their respective boards attempting to toss and catch a bean bag back and forth. When they reach the middle of their boards (about side by side), they perform a half turn and walk backwards to the end of their boards, but still continue to play catch with the bean bag.

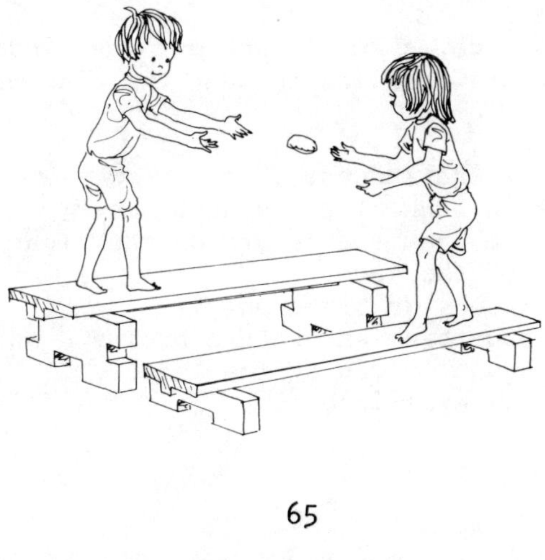

LADDER CHALLENGES

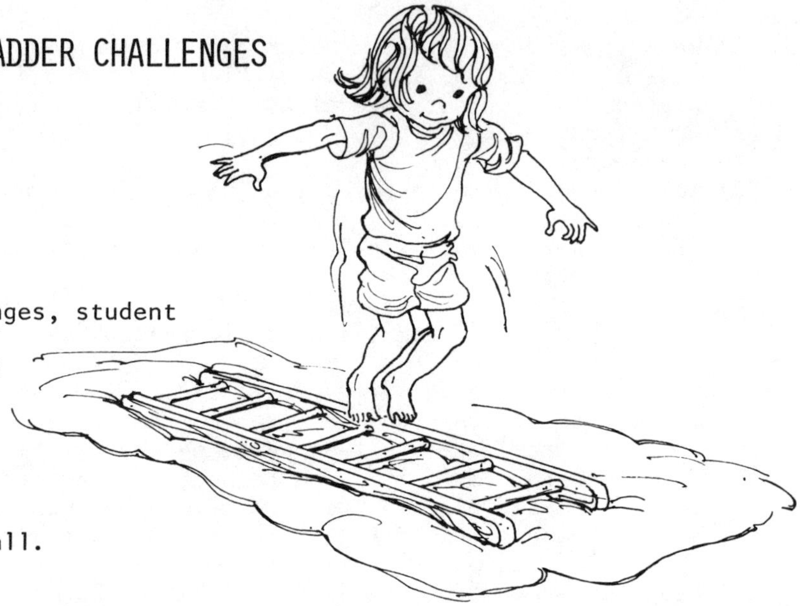

PERFORMANCE OBJECTIVES

By performing the following challenges, student demonstrates gross-motor control, laterality, directionality, spatial orientation, balance, efficient motor planning, and eye-hand and eye-foot coordination.

EQUIPMENT

Coordination ladder and a rubber ball.

GENERAL INFORMATION

The coordination ladder, which is a portable piece of equipment, provides the teacher with a great degree of flexibility in presenting children with purposeful movement experiences. Challenges can easily be adapted to the ability level of all children regardless of their age or grade level.

SAFETY PRECAUTIONS

1) For greater safety, it is best to use mats or carpeting under the ladder.
2) For most movement tasks it is best to have only one student on the ladder at a time.
3) Students should be cautioned to move only as fast as they are able to maintain complete control over their bodies.
4) Do not allow the students to move with just socks on. Either have the shoes on or bare feet. Bare feet provide better tactile stimulation, but stubbing of toes can be a problem with some students.
5) It is *not* advisable to use challenges in which the students must hop or jump *backwards* over and between the rungs of the ladder.

LOCOMOTOR CHALLENGES

1) Walk between rungs of the ladder.
2) Run between the rungs of the ladder.
3) Jump between the rungs of the ladder.
4) Hop between the rungs of the ladder.
5) Alternate jumping and hopping.
6) Use above movements in various patterns:
    a) Every other space.
    b) Forward, sideways, etc.
7) With ladder resting on one side, crawl in and out the windows.
8) Alternate forward and backward crawling through the windows.

BALANCE CHALLENGES

1) Walk forward on the rungs of the ladder.
2) Walk forward with one foot on each of the side beams.
3) Walk forward on the left side beam and return on the right side beam.
4) Walk backward on the rungs of the ladder.
5) Walk backward with the feet on side beams only.
6) Walk backward on the left side beam and return backward on the right side beam.
7) Walk sideways using the rungs or sides of the ladder.
8) Use combinations of the above experiences.

ANIMAL MOVEMENT CHALLENGES

1) Dog walk (using hands and feet):
   a) On rungs of the ladder.
   b) Between the rungs of the ladder.
   c) On the sides of the ladder.
2) Bear walk (moving one side of the body at a time):
   a) On the rungs of the ladder.
   b) Between the rungs of the ladder.
   c) On the sides of the ladder.
3) Crab walk (inverted body position on hands and feet):
   a) On the rungs of the ladder.
   b) Between the rungs of the ladder.
   c) On the sides of the ladder.
4) Rabbit hop (move hands and then feet from a squat position):
   a) Between rungs of the ladder.
   b) Use rungs and spaces between the rungs.
5) Frog jump (push off with hands and feet at the same time from a squat position) between the rungs of the ladder.

CREATIVE EXPLORATION CHALLENGES

1) Show me a different way of jumping through the ladder.
2) Can you move the length of the ladder using only 3 parts of your body for support?
3) How would you move over the ladder like a snake?
4) Who can criss-cross their feet as they move through the ladder?
5) How can you move your body over the ladder without touching the ladder or the spaces between the rungs?

The above 5 items represent just a sampling of the types of problem solving tasks which can be presented to the students.

BALL CHALLENGES

1) Walk on the sides of the ladder and bounce and catch the ball between the rungs.
2) Walk on the rungs of the ladder and bounce and catch the ball between the rungs.
3) Toss and catch the ball while performing the above tasks. Add a toss, clap hands, and catch the ball.
4) Dribble the ball between the rungs while walking on the outside of the ladder. (This is an advanced skill.)
5) Jump over the rungs like a kangaroo with the ball held between the knees.

Note: When working with ball skills, the ladder must be placed on a surface which allows the ball to bounce properly.

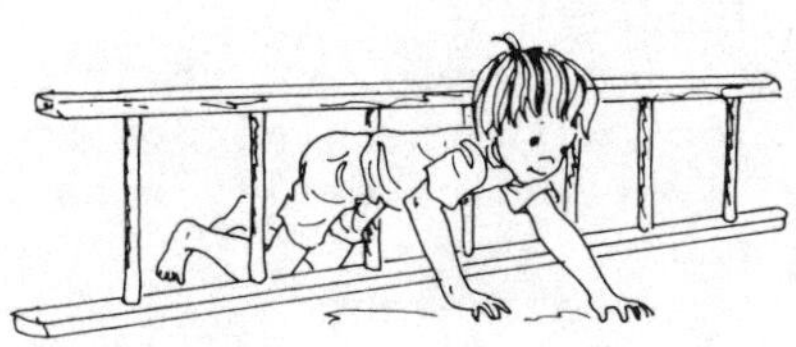

JUMP BOX CHALLENGES

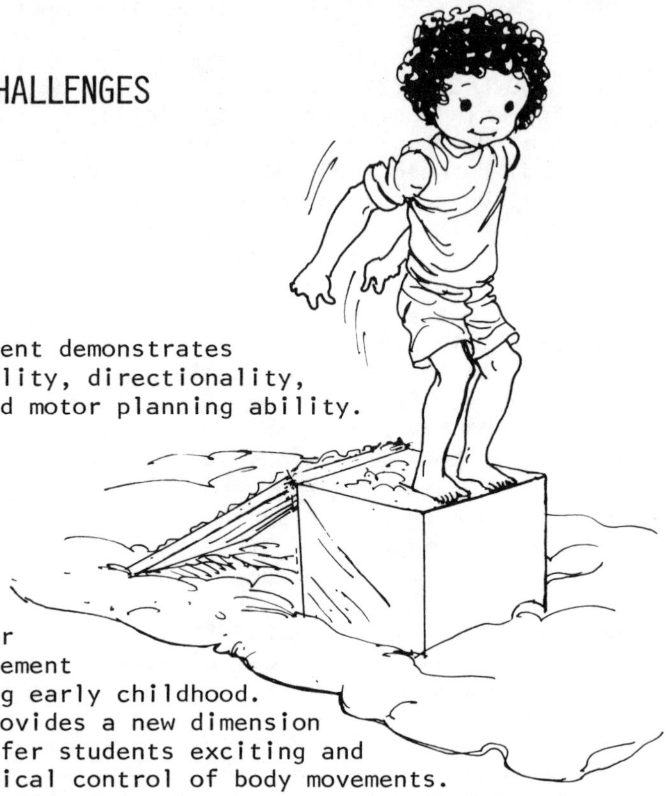

PERFORMANCE OBJECTIVES

By performing the following challenges, student demonstrates balance, space awareness, body image, laterality, directionality, foot-eye coordination, locomotor control, and motor planning ability.

EQUIPMENT

Jump box with incline board, mats, tires, coordination ladder and 2 cross bars.

GENERAL INFORMATION

The ability to jump from various heights and land with complete body control whithout fear of falling or hurting oneself is a basic movement skill which all students should master during early childhood. The jump box with attaching incline board provides a new dimension to movement programs enabling teachers to offer students exciting and fun-filled challenges with the focus on physical control of body movements. Various size boxes or benches may be used to jump from, but in general, a height of approximately 20 inches is an appropriate challenge for most students. The addition of the attaching incline board allows the student to jump from the box after a short run up the board. Construction plans for making a jump box with incline board are included at the end of this book. However, teachers may use any sturdy box or bench to provide most of the basic suggested tasks.

TEACHING SUGGESTIONS

1) The height of the jumping surface is an important consideration in planning your challenges. For emotional security it is best to start at a low level and work up to higher levels as the students gain in skill and self-confidence.
2) Some students will require physical contact at first (holding their hands, etc.) to get them over their initial fear of height.
3) Students should participate in their bare feet so that a better "feel" is acquired for the movements.
4) Mats or carpeting should be used as a landing surface, if the activity takes place indoors or on a hard surface.
5) Long lines of students waiting their turn is self-defeating in that involvement is limited. Use the jump box as one of several learning stations so that opportunities for many repetitions are provided.
6) Obstacles such as bicycle tires (or hoops) and traffic cones with adjustable cross tubes (cross bars) should be used along with the jump box to provide greater challenge and skill development. Old bike tires can be easily spray painted various colors for additional motivation and visual cues.
7) Remember, although the jump box is a tremendous catalyst for movement experiences, the teacher must still teach correct techniques in order for the student to derive maximum benefits from its use.

SAFETY FIRST

1) A carpeted surface on the jump box and incline board prevents students from slipping.
2) Students should be instructed to jump *out* from the box so that if their balance is lost they will not risk falling against the box.

3) Adequate space must be provided so that freedom for safe movement is not curtailed.
4) Only one student should be allowed on the jump box at a time.
5) Students should be taught to bend their knees upon impact with the landing surface so that they lower their center of gravity for greater control and balance.
6) Jumping backwards off the box is a questionable task due to the fact that balance is easily lost and bad falls can result.

SKILLS TO STRESS

1) Stress that a correct starting position with the feet about shoulder distance apart and toes up to the edge of the box be assumed before the jump is made from a stationary position. Both feet should leave the box at the same time on a jump.
2) If movement starts with a run up the incline board, then it is more natural for students to leap from the box with one foot leading. This can be refined into a jump after freedom to leap is explored.
3) Knees should be bent on take-off and landing.
4) Arms are thrust forward and up on take-off to guide and project movement.
5) Feet push off from the top of the box not from the sides which means toes do *not* overhang the top surface of the box.
6) A jump, leap, and a hop are 3 specific locomotor (transport) movements.
   a) On a jump, both feet leave the box at the same time and contact the landing surface at the same time.
   b) On a leap, one foot leads and the other follows.
   c) On a hop from the box, the take-off and landing is made on the same foot with the weight balanced on one foot.
7) Landings are made "softly" on the front part of the feet. *No* flat footed landings!
8) The arms are used to help control and apply "breaks" to the movement upon landing. They should be pulled down low and back near sides of body as impact of feet is made with the landing surface.

CHALLENGES

All tasks listed should be first attempted from a stationary position on the box. Once mastered from a stationary position, a run can be added, if an attaching incline board is available.

1) Jump forward from the box and land with good control and balance. Both feet leave the box at the same time and land at the same time.
2) Jump forward and land in a red bicycle tire used as a target. Tire serves to confine the movement and refine the skill. Red means "stop" and control your body inside the tire.
3) Jump forward and land in one of the 3 bicycle tires placed end to end. Student has a choice of targets and determines own challenge in terms of distance.
4) Jump forward and land with one foot in each of 2 bicycle tires placed side by side and then continue jumping through the tire pattern.
5) Jump forward and over a cross bar (use plastic tube suspended across 2 traffic cones) and land with good control.
6) Jump forward over a cross bar and land in the red tire.

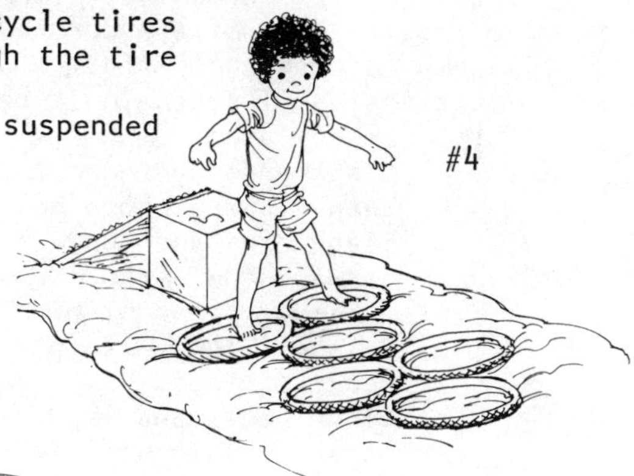
#4

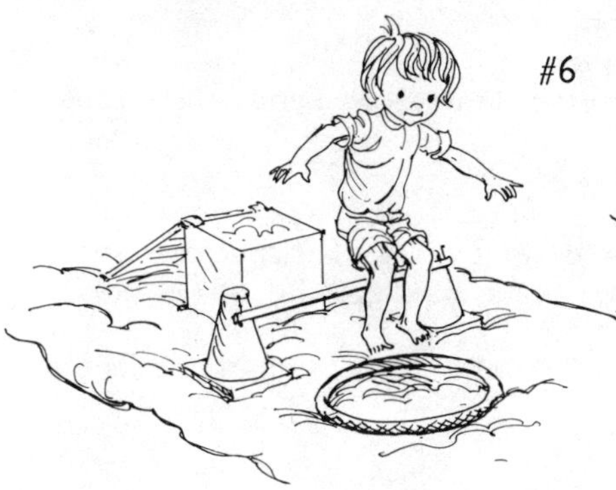
#6

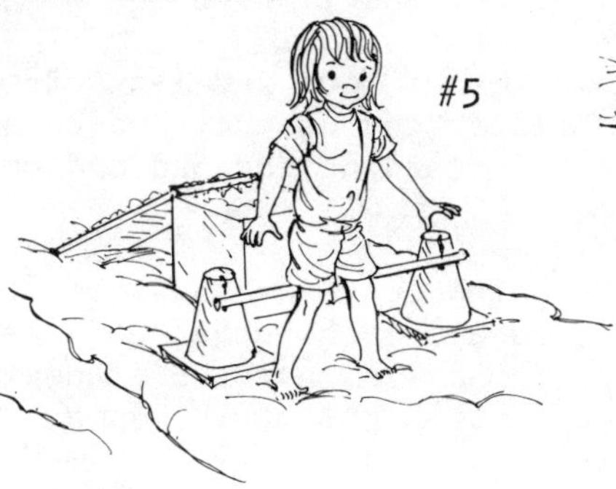
#5

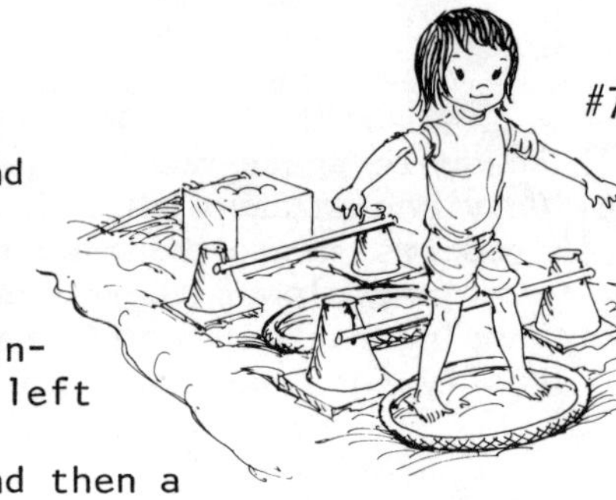

#7

7) Jump forward over a cross bar, land in the red tire, and then jump over a 2nd cross bar and land in the tire.
8) Jump sideways from the box with the right side leading and then with the left side leading.
9) Jump sideways from the box and land in the red tire. Instructor should challenge the student to lead with the left side or right side.
10) Jump forward and perform a quarter turn to the right and then a quarter turn to the left. Emphasize that the turn is made in space after jumping out forward.
11) Same challenge as #10 above using quarter turns, only instructor gives verbal challenge to each student just before the jump is made: "right turn", or "left turn".
12) Jump forward and perform a quarter turn using bicycle tires placed side by side as targets for feet to land in. Use verbal challenges: "right turn", or "left turn".

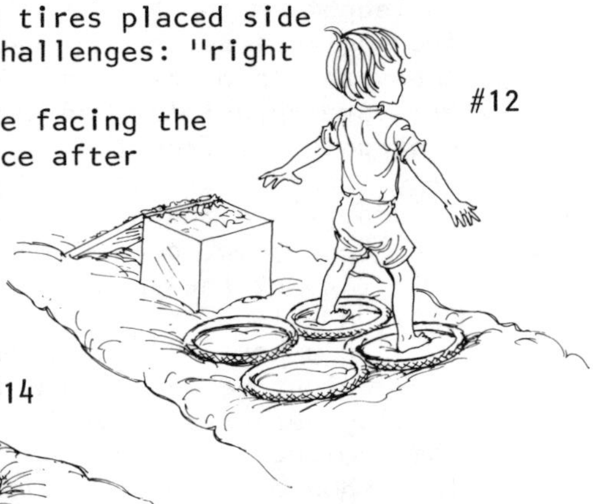

#12

13) Jump forward and perform a half turn with landing made facing the box. Emphasize that the turn or twist is made in space after a forward jump from the box.
14) Jump forward, perform a half turn and land in the bicycle tires placed side by side. One foot lands in each tire with body facing box.

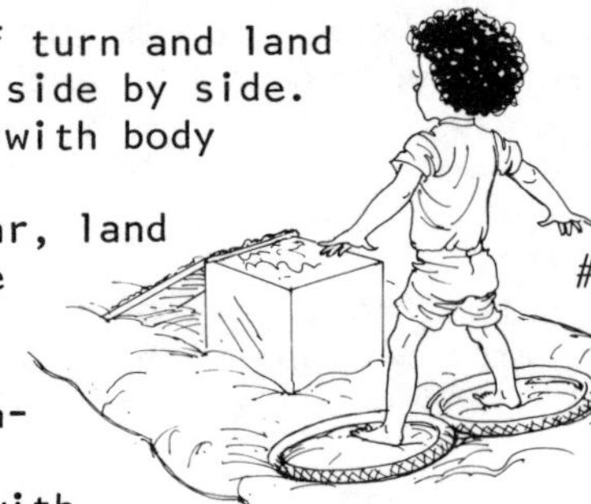

#14

15) Jump forward over a cross bar, land in the red tire and continue through the obstacle course going *under* a cross bar and then *through* a car tire without touching the obstacles.
16) Jump forward, land on feet with good control, and then perform a forward roll. Technique of a forward roll must be taught before this task is presented to the student.

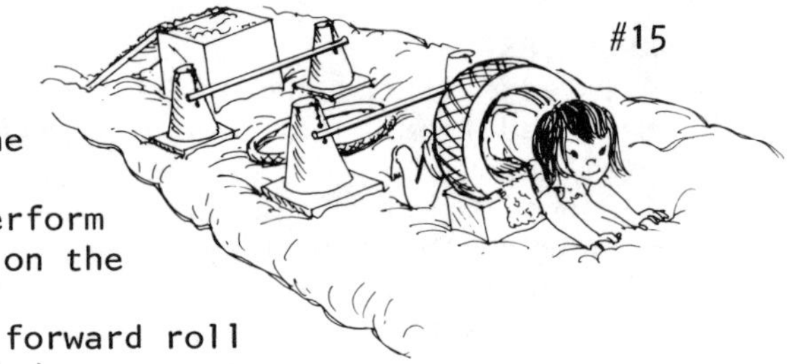

#15

17) Jump forward, land in the bicycle tire and then perform a forward roll out of the tire. Hands are placed on the mat outside of the tire to begin the roll.
18) Jump forward, land in the bicycle tire, perform a forward roll over the low cross bar, and then crawl under the 2nd cross bar without touching. Tire is placed close to the first cross bar with hands placed on the opposite side of the bar to begin the roll.

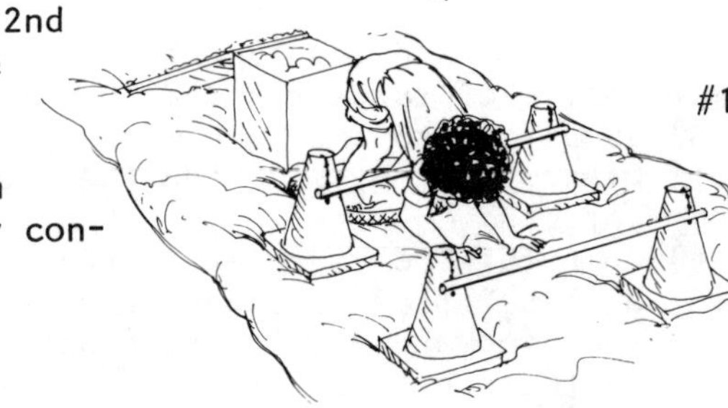

#18

19) Jump forward and perform a series of hand and arm actions as listed below. Land with complete body control and balance.
    a) Clap hands overhead and land.
    b) Snap fingers above head level and land.
    c) Slap knees and land.
20) Jump forward and perform a series of foot and leg actions as listed below. Land with complete body control and balance.
    a) Scissors jump with one foot leading forward and one backwards. Land with legs back together.
    b) Click heels and land.
    c) Straddle jump with legs going out wide and then land with legs back together.
21) Jump forward from the box, grab a 7 inch rubber ball held up by the instructor and land with the ball in hand. Emphasize that the student jumps out to the ball and attempts to grasp the ball at the height of the jump.
22) Hop forward from the box (weight on one foot) and land with the body supported and

balanced on the take-off foot. Student that is successful on the preferred foot should be challenged to use the opposite foot.

23) Hop forward from the box and land on one foot inside the red bicycle tire. Use a small tire to confine the space and refine the skill.

24) Use the coordination ladder, if available, and attach (support) on top of the jump box. Challenge the student to move up the ladder in various ways and jump from the box. Use obstacles (tires or cross bar) as in previous tasks to add to the challenge.

25) Use a coordination ladder with a jump box and an incline board. Challenge the student to move up the ladder in various ways and then go down the incline board. To add difficulty to the movements, challenge the student to go up the incline board first, and then down the ladder in various ways. A wide variety of challenges can be used in different combinations or sequences.

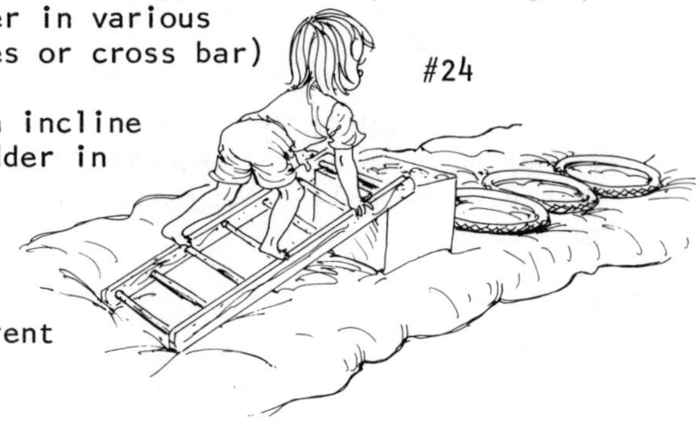

#24

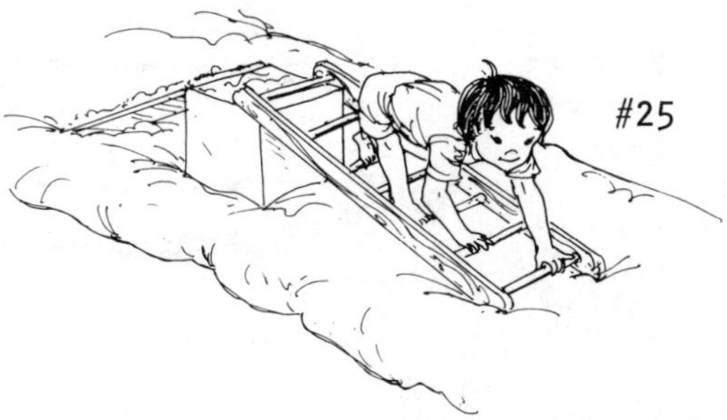

#25

REBOUNDER CHALLENGES

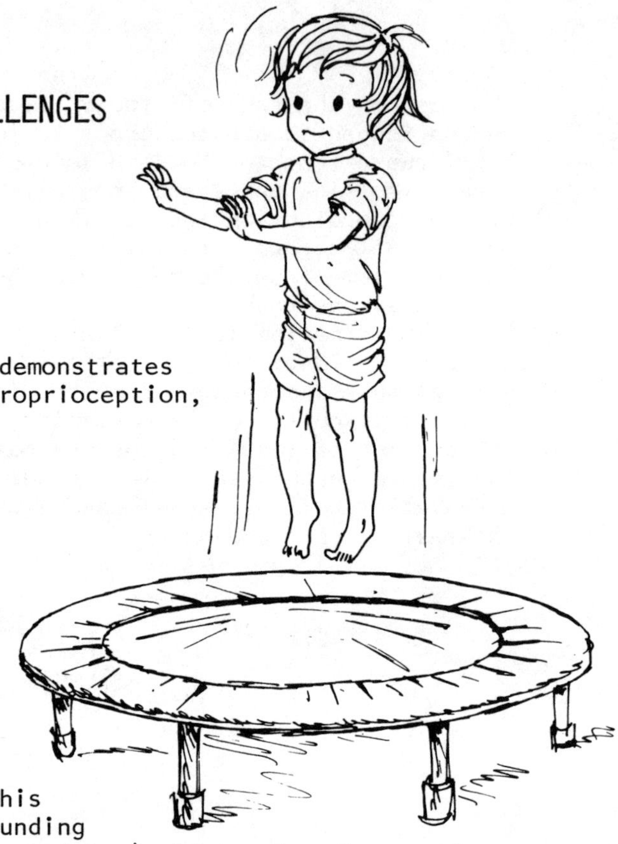

PERFORMANCE OBJECTIVES

By performing the following challenges, student demonstrates balance, laterality, body and space awareness, proprioception, and locomotor control.

EQUIPMENT

Rebounder and mats.

GENERAL INFORMATION

The "rebounder" represents an exciting and challenging piece of equipment designed for safe use by preschool, kindergarten, and primary grade children as well as older age groups. It is excellent for developing muscular control and coordination as well as general body fitness. The rebounder is *not* classified as a trampoline, therefore, most insurance companies will cover this equipment item for liability purposes. All rebounding is performed on the feet in an upright (standing position) which makes for continuous safe use. Due to the "nature" of this piece of equipment, it *does* require close supervision and careful attention to basic rules as outlined in this section.

ORGANIZATION REMINDERS

1) Before allowing any child to perform on the rebounder, carefully review the basic safety rules with the entire class.
2) Due to the fact that the rebounder is designed and constructed for use by just one child at a time, it should normally be used as a station activity. Those children waiting their turn are lined up around the rebounder and serve as "spotters".
3) If mats are available, it is best for extra safety to place mats on the floor around the rebounder.
4) The children should remove their shoes and socks before being allowed on the rebounder.
5) There is *no* weight limit for using the rebounder. It is very durable!

SAFETY RULES

1) Short turns are important! Long turns can lead to accidents, as the child becomes tired, particularly the legs, before he/she realizes it.
2) Encourage children to rebound (jump) only in the center of the matting.
3) Discourage high rebounding (jumping). *Good control is the most important factor!*
4) Do *not* allow children to jump off the rebounder onto the floor. The child should carefully step down. (The legs are affected by continous jumping on the matting and will *not* always control the body when landing on a hard surface.)
5) Only one child is allowed on the rebounder at a time.
6) Do *not* tolerate any "horseplay". Insist that children only attempt stunts that are presented in the lessons. There is no room for show-offs!
7) Use "spotters" around the rebounder and explain to "spotters" that they must be alert and help to keep the jumper on the rebounder, if balance is lost.

8) Never force a child to do a stunt, if they have not mastered previous stunts, or if they are overly fearful.
9) Always place (turn) the rebounder up on ends against a wall when not in use.
10) All stunts are performed in an upright position. Stunts such as seat drops, knee drops, flips, etc., are *not* allowed on this equipment item.
11) Make sure the rebounder is placed on a level surface when in use.
12) Never allow any child to be on the rebounder unless it is supervised by a qualified adult.

INSTRUCTIONS FOR REBOUNDING

1) Child should assume a starting position over the center of the canvas bed with feet placed apart approximately the width of the shoulders.
2) Eyes focus on the instructor (or a focus point) *not* down at the feet or around the room.
3) Discourage flat-footed rebounding. Child should push off from toes and "balls" of feet.
4) Unbalanced landings or take-offs are the chief danger. Emphasize fully-controlled rebounding at a low level.
5) The "natural" give in the legs and knees when landing is used to "kill" (stop) movement. This should be the first skill taught.
6) In rebounding, the body stays fairly straight and firm to allow for a balanced movement except for the "kill" as mentioned in #5 above.
7) For jumping vertically (rebounding), the head and trunk must be kept in alignment, if the jumper is to go up straight with good control.
8) Arms are used in front of the body when jumping. However, it should be noted that excessive arm action tends to disturb balance rather than helping.
9) It is vital that the jumper is always aware of the position of his/her body in relation to the center of the canvas bed. The child attempts to always take-off and land in approximately the same spot near the center of the bed.
10) The height of the jump (rebound) is controlled largely by the extension of the ankles.

SUGGESTED BASIC PROGRESSION OF TASKS

1) Heel bounces (toes stay in contact with matting).
2) Cross-lateral marching (walking in place over center point of matting). (Note that "cross-lateral" refers to opposition of limb movement, that is, left arm with right leg and right arm with left leg.)
3) Cross-lateral jogging (running in place over center spot with high knee action and opposition of limb movement).
4) Controlled rebounding (jumping with feet apart).
    a) Start with feet approximately shoulder distance apart over center area of matting.
    b) Students take 5 jumps and freeze (stop). Repeat.
5) Controlled rebounding with quarter turns.
    a) Use rhythmic count 1-2-turn, etc. (Student rebounds 2 times and performs quarter turn, etc.)
    b) Four quarter turns return student to starting position.
6) Controlled rebounding with half turns.
    a) Use rhythmic count 1-2-turn, etc.
    b) Two half turns will return the student to starting position.
7) Straddle jumping (rebounding).
    a) Start with feet close over center point (may wish to have hands placed on hips).
    b) Student jumps with feet moving apart out to sides and then back to starting position.
8) Lateral (side) jumping.
    a) Start with feet *together* over center point.
    b) Student jumps in short sideward movements with feet staying together.
    c) "Spot" this task carefully. Student can easily lose control.
9) Hopping (preferred foot).
    a) Start with weight on one foot over center point.
    b) Student attempts to control movement for a series of 3 to 5 hops.

10) Hopping (opposite foot).
11) Alternate hopping (2-2 rhythm).
    a) Start on preferred foot and hop 2 times, then switch to opposite foot and hop 2 times.
    b) Rhythmic hopping pattern continues.
12) Jumping jacks.
    a) Start with feet together over center point and arms down at sides.
    b) Hands and arms go out and up over head as feet jump out to sides, then back to starting position. Rhythmic pattern continues.
13) Front kicks. Alternate feet kick forward with legs kept fairly straight.
14) Side kicks. Alternate feet kick sideward with legs kept fairly straight.
15) Rebounding with ball catching. Student jumps and catches ball thrown underhand by teacher or aide. Student tosses ball back to teacher or aide, and attempts to maintain rhythmic rebounding.
16) Rebounding with net tossing.
    a) Student jumps and tosses bean bag or ball against rebound (pitch back) net which is placed on the floor a short distance from the rebounder.
    b) Student attempts to catch bean bag (or ball) while continuing rhythmic jumping.
17) Rebounding with rope jumping.
    a) Students attempt to jump rope while rebounding.
    b) This is an advanced stunt which many students will not be ready for.
    c) Only allow students with good motor coordination to attempt this stunt.

SENSORIMOTOR TASKS

The tasks listed below may be introduced at any point after basic controlled rebounding has been mastered.

1) Auditory Rebounding
    a) Teacher or aide stands behind student who is on rebounder and bounces a rubber ball a given number of times. (Student does *not* see instructor.)
    b) Student must listen carefully and jump the number of times that the ball has been bounced.
2) Tactile Rebounding
    a) Teacher or aide stands behind student who is on the rebounder, and using a finger, writes (transcribes) a number on the student's back.
    b) Student attempts to jump the same number of times as the number written on his/her back.
3) Visual Response Rebounding
    a) Teacher or aide holds up a flash card with arrow pointing in a given direction. (Examples: Up, Down, Left, Right, etc. ⟶ .) Student must call out correct direction while maintaining rhythmic jumping pattern.
    b) Teacher or aide holds up a flash card with geometric shape (circle, square, etc.) pictured on the card. Student must call out correct shape.
    c) Visual flash cards may also be used with numbers, letters, words, etc.
4) Numbers Rebounding
    a) Teacher or aide verbally gives the student a math problem (example: 2 + 3). Student must jump the correct answer. (5 jumps.)
    b) Teacher or aide holds up a flash card with math problem. Student must jump the answer.
5) Body Awareness Rebounding--Teacher or aide calls out body part and student must touch that body part while continuing to rebound in a rhythmic pattern. (Example: Shoulders or hips.)

IMPORTANT TEACHING SUGGESTION

It is normally a good idea to have students review and practice tasks from a standing position on the floor before attempting the tasks on the rebounder. This can be accomplished as a group rather than individual practice sessions.

GEOMETRIC SHAPE CHALLENGES

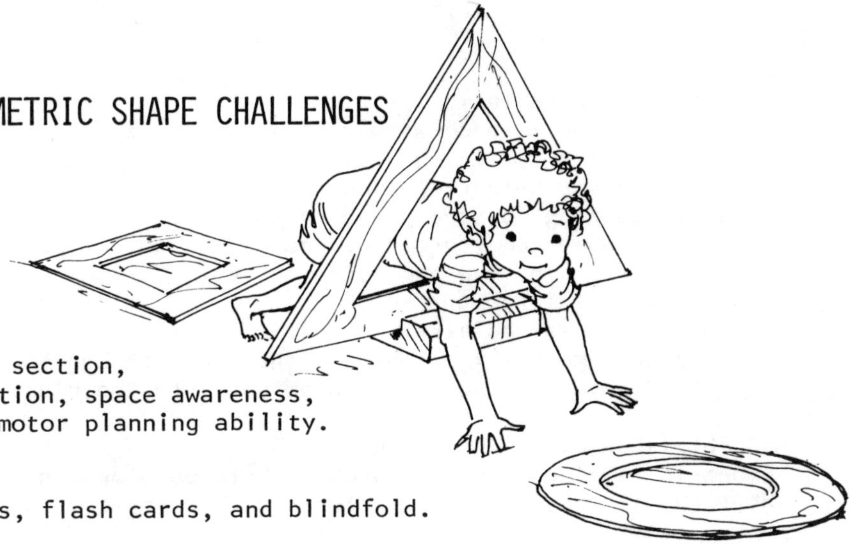

PERFORMANCE OBJECTIVES

By performing challenges in this section, student demonstrates form perception, space awareness, auditory memory sequencing, and motor planning ability.

EQUIPMENT

Classroom set of geometric shapes, flash cards, and blindfold.

GENERAL INFORMATION

The basic set of geometric shapes consists of 8 shapes of 2 circles, 2 squares, 2 rectangles, and 2 triangles along with support stands for each individual shape. Plywood is used to make the shapes and it is possible to cut 2 shapes (large and small) out of each sheet of plywood except for the triangle. The shapes are painted with 4 colors: red, blue, green, and yellow. The shapes may be used by placing them upright in their support stands, or by placing them flat on the floor.

CREATIVE EXPLORATION CHALLENGES

Students are asked to explore all the shapes from a creeping position and see how many different shapes they can discover as well as different sizes and colors.

VERBAL CHALLENGES

Visual recognition along with auditory memory sequencing are combined using basic shape, size, and color as an integral part of the challenges.

1) Use Of Shape - Can you move through a triangle? (Square, circle, rectangle.)
2) Use Of Size - Can you move through the largest or smallest of a specific shape?
3) Use Of Color - Who can move through a green rectangle and then through a blue square?
4) Use Of Structure - Who can go through a shape with 4 equal sides?
5) Use Of Dimension - Who can go through the narrowest shape?

VISUAL FLASH CARD CHALLENGES

Cards showing either a circle, square, rectangle, or triangle are held up for a few moments and then the student must respond to the visual cues presented. No auditory cues are used in this method.

TACTILE BLINDFOLDED CHALLENGES

Students wear blindfolds when it is their turn to be challenged. They are placed in a creeping position and asked to feel each shape they come in contact with, identify it, and go through it.

MOVEMENT SEQUENCING WITH SHAPES FLAT ON THE FLOOR CHALLENGES

1) Students are verbally challenged to perform basic locomotor skills either inside a shape or on a shape. Some examples follow.
   a) Show me how you can jump 3 times inside the largest circle, then hop 2 times inside the largest square.
   b) Try jumping from the circle into the triangle.
   c) Can you perform a toe-heel balance walk on the red rectangle? Walk completely around it.

2) Static Balance Tasks
   a) Can you balance with 2 body parts inside a square and 2 body parts inside a rectangle?
   b) Can you balance on one foot inside a yellow triangle?
3) Ball Bouncing Tasks
   a) Show me how you can bounce and catch the ball 4 times inside the largest circle.
   b) Can you bounce and catch the ball 2 times inside a small square and 3 times inside a large triangle?
4) Bean Bag Tossing Tasks
   a) Show me how you can toss the red bean bag into a red circle, etc.
   b) Can you toss the blue bean bag into the blue rectangle? Etc.

LANGUAGE (VOCABULARY) CHALLENGES

Emphasis is placed on key words to help develop language concepts such as "through", "between", "over", "into", "closest", "farthest", "smallest", "largest", etc.

NUMBER CONCEPT CHALLENGES

Focus is on awareness of numbers, quantity, etc.
1) Can you move through 1 shape?
2) Who can move through 4 different shapes?
3) Can you move through "more" shapes than the child before?
4) How would you move through "less than" the child before?

SET CONCEPT CHALLENGES

Focus is on requiring child to sort and identify likenesses.
1) Can you move through a set of shapes with straight lines?
2) Can you move through the set of small shapes?
3) Move through the set of shapes with curved sides.

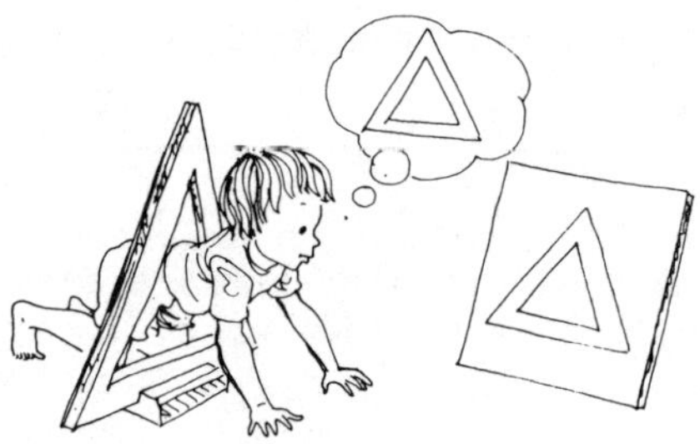

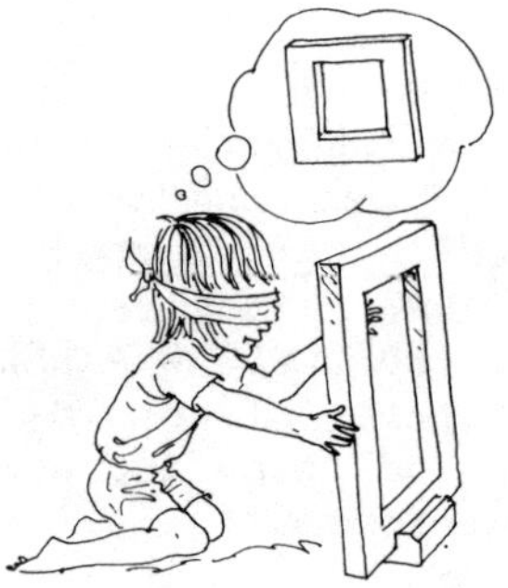

BALANCE PUZZLE CHALLENGES

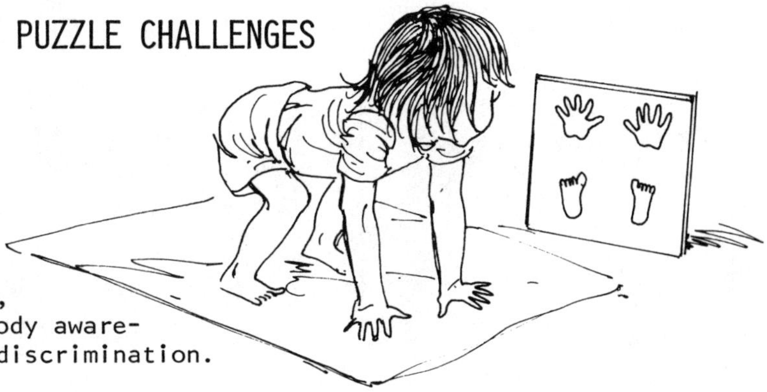

PERFORMANCE OBJECTIVES
By performing the following challenges, student demonstrates static balance, body awareness, spatial orientation, and visual discrimination.

EQUIPMENT
Plastic floor runner (plastic sheet), red, blue, green, and yellow self-adhesive contact paper. Other equipment for alternate uses would be a blackboard with chalk or large chart paper or flash cards. (See sample patterns of "Suggested Balance Puzzles" on page 78.)

GENERAL INFORMATION
The use of balance puzzles in the physical education program can be an exciting and fun experience which will lead to improvement in basic perceptual-motor abilities. The puzzles offer challenges which will help students to develop better control and awareness of their body in space. Students are encouraged to think and solve balance problems within their own ability level.

Ask the students to spread out in the available space so that they have enough room to balance on various body parts without interfering with others. Starting with easier puzzles such as puzzle #1 of the sample patterns of the "Suggested Balance Puzzles" shown on page 78, hold up one puzzle at a time and ask students to balance on body parts as illustrated in the puzzle. They must balance with correct parts (left or right) as well as in the same position as shown with *no other body parts touching the floor*.

PARTNER ROTATION CHALLENGES
Spread out individual puzzles around the available space and assign 2 students (partners) to each puzzle. There will be a few extra puzzles depending on the size of the class. On the signal to begin, one student at each balance puzzle attempts to solve the problem by balancing with the correct body parts. Each partner should be given the opportunity to solve the balance problem before a signal is given to move on to the next number. Partners move together from puzzle to puzzle until completing all the puzzles. 15 to 20 puzzles will keep an entire class active for a full 20 to 30 minutes.

OBSTACLE COURSE CHALLENGES
Use the puzzles as a part of an obstacle course. When students arrive at a puzzle, they must perform the designated balance task before moving onto the next obstacle.

SCRAMBLE CHALLENGES
Puzzles are spread out around the available space with one or 2 students assigned to each puzzle. Each student assumes the balance position as indicated on the puzzle. When the signal (whistle) is given, they must quickly move (scramble) to a new puzzle and assume the position of balance. Students hold balance position until signal is given to scramble. Each time the whistle signal is given, all participants attempt to find a new puzzle.

SUGGESTED BALANCE PUZZLES

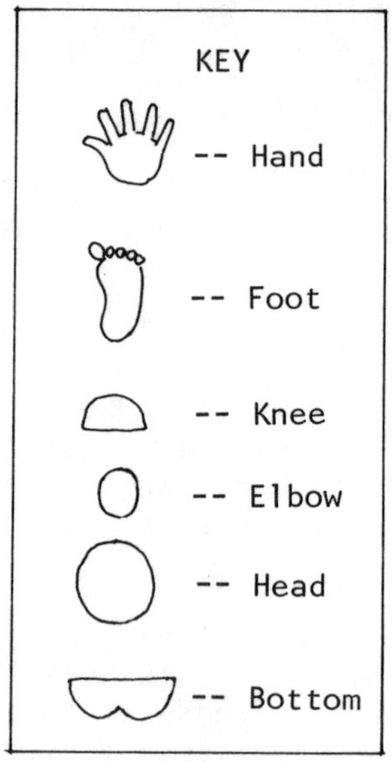

COLORS

Blue	-- Left
Red	-- Right
Green	-- Head
Yellow	-- Bottom

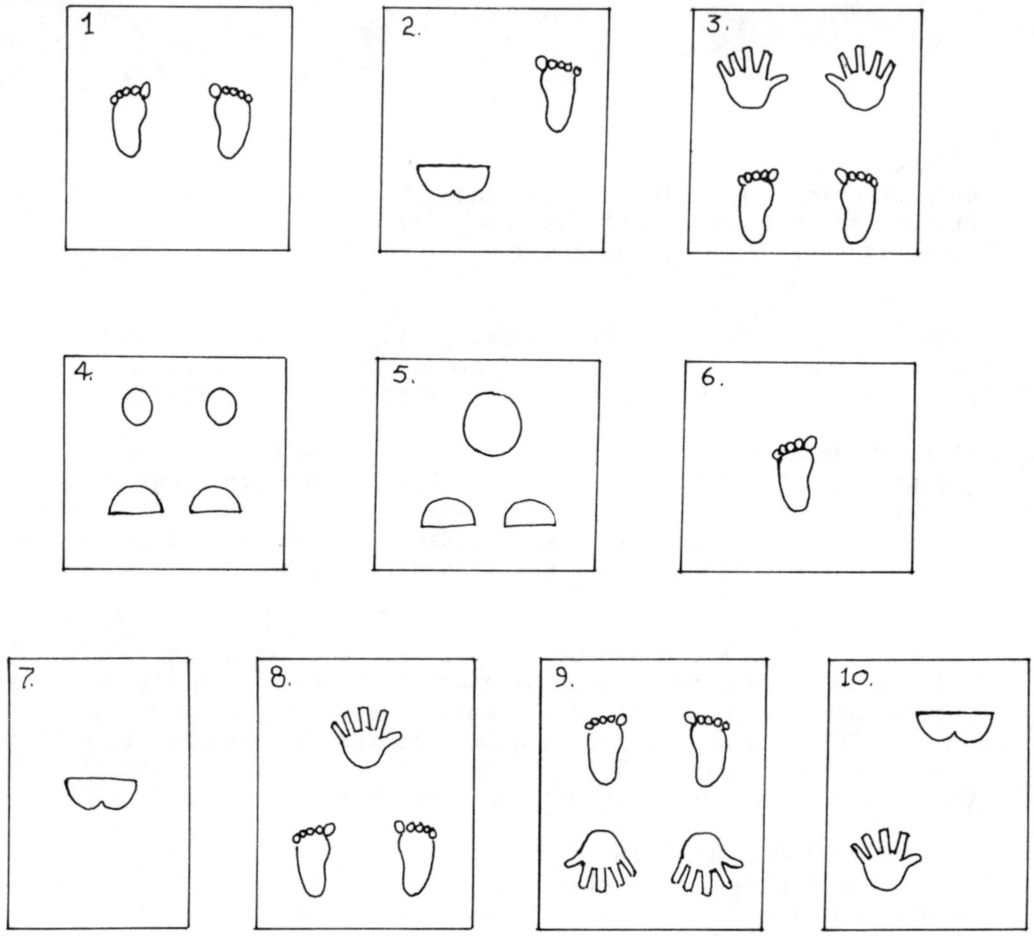

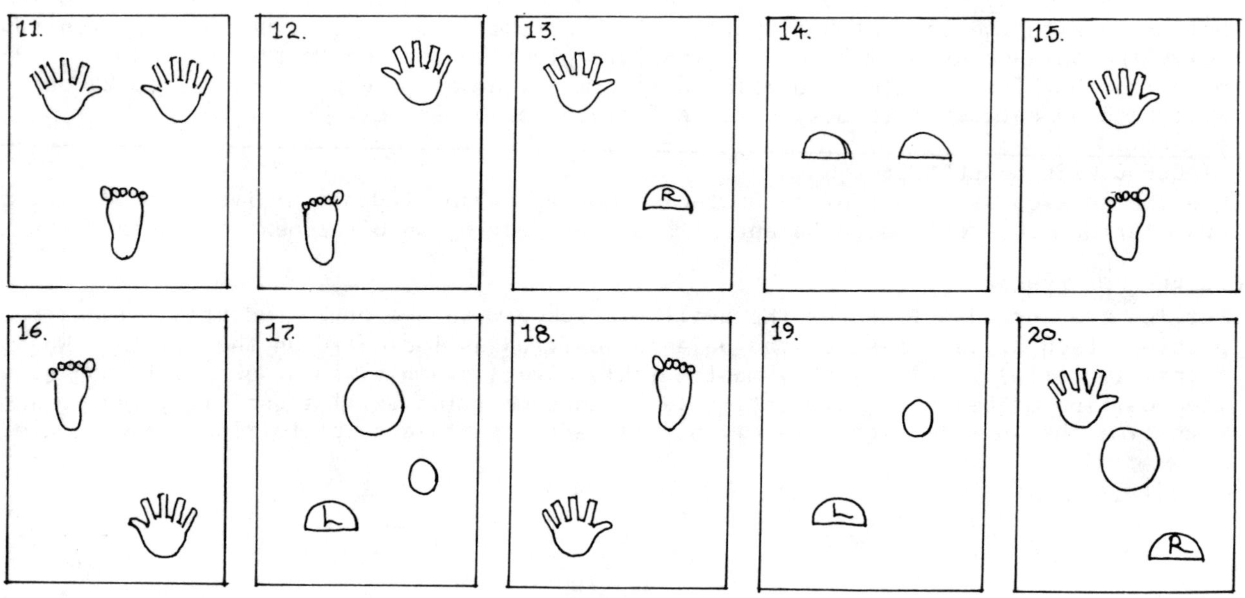

MAT CHALLENGES

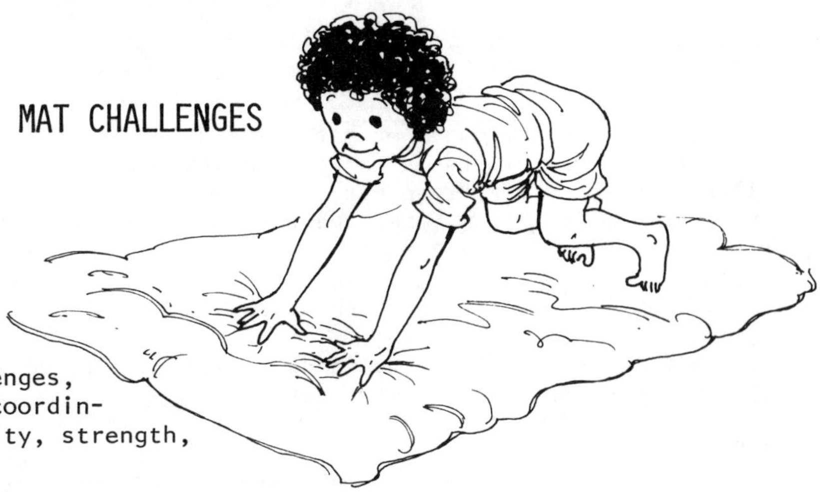

PERFORMANCE OBJECTIVES

By performing the following challenges, student demonstrates gross motor coordination, balance, flexibility, agility, strength, and spatial orientation.

EQUIPMENT

Classroom set of mats.

GENERAL INFORMATION

Students need to be exposed to movement experiences in which maximum stress is placed on body control and management. Many of these types of experiences which offer lasting values to students, place them in a position on their back or stomach, or involves them in rolling, crawling, and jumping type actions. It therefore becomes necessary to incorporate the use of mats into your program. This will help to assure that proper safety precautions are exercised, will give protection to clothing, and also serve to enhance the participants degree of self-confidence. The teacher should not have a fear of conducting mat activities, keeping in mind that you gear the activity to the level and ability of your students. A major point to remember is that students must feel comfortable in doing stunts which they are asked to perform. Simple individual movement challenges can be the foundation of a very purposeful mat activity program. This approach leads to success experiences for all students, not just the well coordinated student.

TEACHING SUGGESTIONS

1) Students remove shoes for mat cleanliness.
2) All movement starts and finishes on the mats.
3) Each student progresses at his/her own rate of speed.
4) Students should never be on the mats without on-the-spot supervision from the teacher.
5) One-way traffic only should be allowed on the mats.
6) For greater involvement, have students work across the width of the mat, as opposed to the length. (This has to be determined in relationship to the type of activity. For example: Animal movements are best performed length-wise for continuous repetition.)
7) Appropriate clothing, especially for girls, is most important.
8) Lessons should begin with warm-up activities.

ANIMAL MOVEMENT CHALLENGES

The student imitates the actions of familiar animals and in the process is learning to use the body with ease and confidence. The lesson will be more meaningful if rhythm instruments are used to maintain a definite beat which each student responds to. Mats are optional.

BEAR WALK

1) Bend over and walk on all 4's.
2) Move one side of the body at the same time. (Left hand and left leg then right hand and right leg.)
3) Walk slowly and keep limbs fairly straight.

RABBIT HOP

1) Squat and place hands on mats *outside* of knees.
2) Place hands forward as far as the student can reach.
3) Keeping both feet together, jump feet to hands.
4) Continue in this movement pattern down the mat.

CRAB WALK

1) Weight is supported on both hands and both feet, with the body facing upward. (Stomach up.)
2) Walk backwards (head and hands first) in this position.
3) Keep hips up and back straight.

FROG JUMP

1) Squat and place hands on mat *inside* the knees.
2) Move forward by jumping on all 4's. (Spring off the floor.)
3) Land on feet first.

KANGAROO HOP

1) Assume squat position, with the arms folded across the chest.
2) Spring from the floor as high as possible and as far forward as possible.
3) Land in squat position with arms folded.

GORILLA WALK

1) Start with feet apart, trunk bent forward slightly, arms hanging loosely in front. (For more challenging method have students grip ankles with hands.)
2) Walk forward imitating a gorilla.
3) Take slow lumbering steps.

ELEPHANT WALK

1) Bend over at the waist, use one hand for the trunk and one for the tail.
2) Swing trunk while walking.
3) Try to swing and swish trunk across the mat surface while walking.

SEAL WALK

1) Place hands on floor under shoulders, elbows stiff and legs stretched (extended) out behind. (Similar to a push-up position.)
2) Ankles are extended back with weight on top of toes and feet. Walk forward with hands, legs, and toes dragging behind.
3) Swing body from side to side.

MAT EXERCISE CHALLENGES

Many valuable physical exercises which do not adapt themselves to the playground setting can be performed with enthusiasm on mats and should become a regular part of your mat program. They can also serve as warm-up activities for other stunts.

SIT-UP

1) Student lies on back with knees bent and feet flat on the floor or mat. Heels are about a foot from the buttocks.
2) Hands are placed back of the neck with fingers clasped and elbows squarely on the mat. A partner may hold the student's ankles.
3) To perform the sit-up, the student brings elbows and head forward as he or she curls up, touching elbows to knees. This action constitutes one sit-up.
4) If this type of sit-up is too difficult for some students, the teacher may give them a modified type. Legs straight is one step in modification, and next would be to allow student to keep the arms out straight and touch fingers to toes.

KNEE PUSH-UP

1) Student kneels on the mat and places hands on mat under shoulders with arms extended.
2) Feet are raised off the mat so that the student is supported only on hands and knees. Body is straight from head to knees.
3) One knee push-up consists of bending the arms and lowering the body until the chest touches the mat and then pushing up again with the arms until they are fully extended.

BICYCLE PUMPING

1) Student lies down on back and lifts both legs so that they are extended (straight up) overhead.
2) The back must be supported with the hands.
3) The legs are then pumped up and down as if peddling a bicycle. (It is not a waving action with the feet.)

ELEVATOR

1) Student begins exercise by sitting on mat with legs extended and hands placed flat on the mat next to the hips.
2) The student pushes against the mat with his or her hands and slowly elevates the trunk and legs up off the mat. The weight is now supported on the hands and heels of the feet.
3) When the body reaches a fully extended position (straight) from head to toes, the student holds this position and then slowly returns to starting position.

TOP SPIN

1) Place feet in stride position on mat. (Shoulder distance apart.)
2) Spring from the floor and swing arms and trunk in the direction the turn is to be made. (Teacher directs first a 1/4 turn and works towards a full turn.) (1/4 turn, 1/2, 3/4, and full turn.)
3) Land with feet in the same stride position.
4) To make it more difficult, require students to keep hands on their hips throughout the exercise.

SIMPLE STUNT CHALLENGES

Simple stunts are ones which present a definite challenge, but are *not* so demanding that students develop fear and are afraid to try them. They allow for good developmental possibilities within their structure and sometimes serve to promote lead-up skills necessary for more complex stunt activities.

EGG SIT

1) Student sits on mat with knees bent close to the chest.
2) Grasp right toe with right hand and left toe with left hand.
3) Rock back on buttocks moving back and forth.

SNAIL

1) Student lies down on back with arms extended at sides and hands flat on the mat.
2) Both legs are lifted so that they will rise overhead and touch the mat behind the head with the toes.
3) Student holds this position and if help is needed to keep balance, the back may be supported with hands.

THREAD THE NEEDLE

1) Student should start by clasping hands in front of the body.
2) Bend trunk forward and step through the clasped hands with the right foot.
3) Follow with the left foot and stand erect with hands clasped in rear of body.
4) Return by stepping backward through the clasped hands, first on one foot, then the other. Stand erect.

HEEL CLICK

1) Student stands erect with feet slightly apart.
2) Spring up in the air and click heels together.
3) Come down with feet apart and the body in a balanced position.
4) Teach students to land lightly on balls of feet with relaxed knees and ankles.

TURK STAND

1) Student stands with arms and legs crossed.
2) Keep the legs crossed and ease into a sitting position. Arms also must remain crossed (folded at chest level).
3) Place weight over feet and rise to a standing position immediately.
4) Keep balance to finish as in starting position, arms and legs still crossed.

LAY OUT AND MACHINE GUN DRILL

1) The student kneels on mat with arms extended, hands flat on mat under shoulders.
2) The back should be kept fairly straight with the head up.
3) On a signal, usually a whistle or hand clap, the student lays out flat on the mat, slapping the mat with the palm of the hands as contact is made.
4) A machine gun reaction drill can be performed by having each student react in order from one end of the mats to the other.

COFFEE GRINDER

1) Student places the heel of one *hand* on the mat with the arm extended. Weight is on the hand and feet.
2) Extend both legs sideward as far as possible.
3) Keeping legs extended, walk around the hand in a complete circle.
4) Try it changing hands and moving in the opposite direction.

FROG HEAD BALANCE

1) Student kneels on mat and assumes a tripod position. (Hands and head form a triangle with the head forward on the mat and the arms placed comfortably a shoulder's width apart on the mat.)
2) Place knees on top of bent elbows and tip up from this position. (Head remains on the mat.)
3) Student balances his or her body in this position.

ROLLING STUNT CHALLENGES

A roll is a stunt in which the body completely changes position in space. This type of activity leads to improved body awareness and spatial orientation. Rolls can be simple or complex in nature. Simple roll experiences which the student can feel comfortable with will meet the needs of primary grade students.

LOG ROLL

1) Student lies across mat in a prone position with arms extended overhead.
2) Body should be straight and firm from head to toes.
3) Roll over and over by rotating shoulders and hips in the direction the turn is to be made. Proceed down the mat in this manner.

EGG ROLL

1) Student kneels across the mat with legs slightly apart and back rounded.
2) Fold arms and rest elbows on mat in front of knees.
3) Push to the side with arms and knees to start the roll.
4) Roll to the side, onto the back, to the other side and up to the original position. This makes a complete roll.

HUMAN BALL

1) Student sits on the mat with knees bent and apart. The ankles should be crossed.
2) Bring the arms down between the legs, then around the outside of the legs, and clasp the hands together in front of the ankles.
3) Start momentum by a slightly swaying motion from side to side. Roll over on side (thigh and shoulders) and continue rolling to back, then opposite side and up again to starting position.
4) In 2 complete rolls a circle is scribed.

FORWARD ROLL

1) Assume a squat position by bending knees and placing toes up to the edge of the mat. Hands are placed on the outside of the legs. (Some students find it easier to perform the roll with hands placed on the inside of the legs.)
2) Bend over until the head almost touches the mat. (The student should now be looking between the legs and hips are in a raised position.)
3) Push off with the toes and roll forward keeping hands in the starting position to support the body. (Back of head, not the top should touch the mat.)

BACKWARD ROLL

1) Student starts with an egg sit keeping knees bent and close to the chest.
2) After squatting and sitting back on the mat, tuck the chin against the chest, pull with the knees and roll back keeping the body in a tight ball.
3) Hands should reach the mat just before the head allowing the body to continue rolling over. (By giving a push upward with hands as the body weight comes over the hands, the starting position can be assumed.)

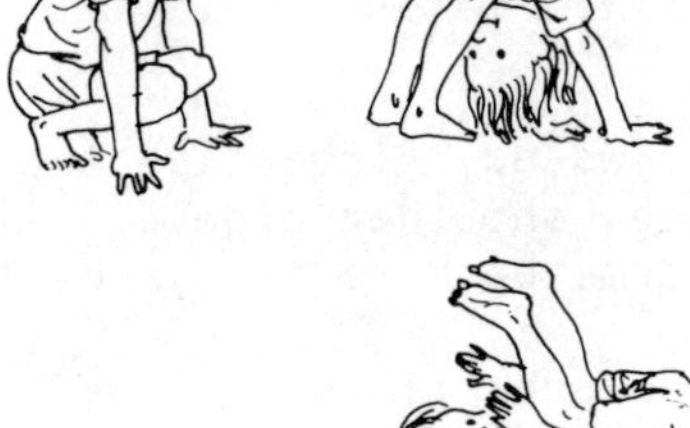

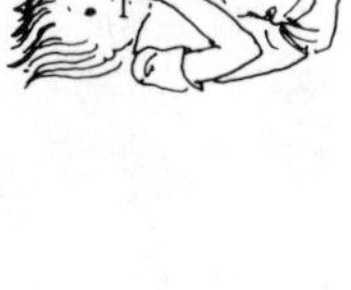

BODY CONDITIONING CHALLENGES

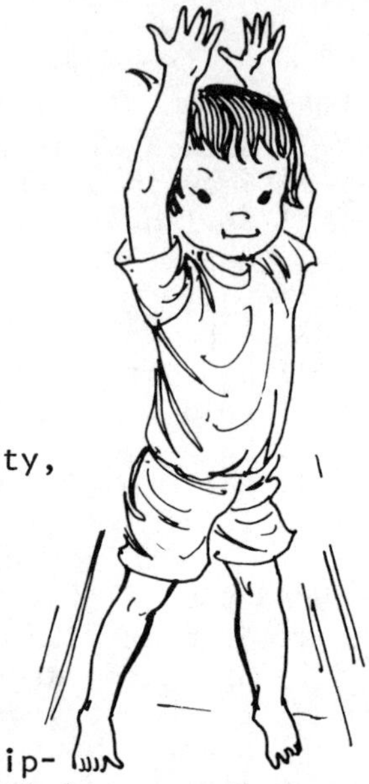

PERFORMANCE OBJECTIVES

By performing the following challenges, student demonstrates flexibility, strength, balance, and gross motor coordination.

EQUIPMENT

None.

GENERAL INFORMATION

Simple conditioning exercises may be performed any time or place, indoors or out, with large groups or small. No specific supplies or equipment are needed, and they are easy to introduce as well as fun for participants. Exercises are normally performed in unison and should be done correctly and with vigor. Either the teacher or a capable student may serve as the leader of the exercises. Not only will these exercises help to condition the muscles of the body, but they also can serve as a refreshing change of pace from quiet sitting or other forms of classroom inactivity.

ARM-SHOULDER DEVELOPMENT CHALLENGES

ARM FLIP-FLOPS

Ready - Take stride position, arms hanging at sides.
Count 1 - Raise arms forcefully over head, shoulders back.
Count 2 - Flop forward at waist, touching hands to feet.

Repeat flipping up and flopping down several times.

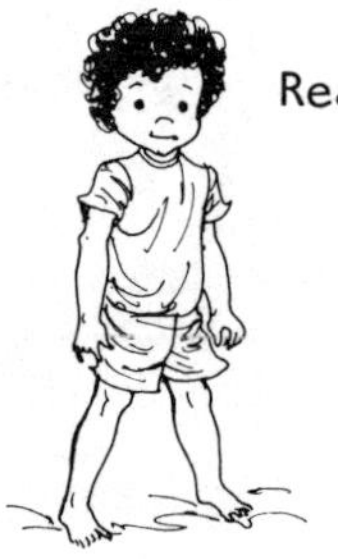

Ready

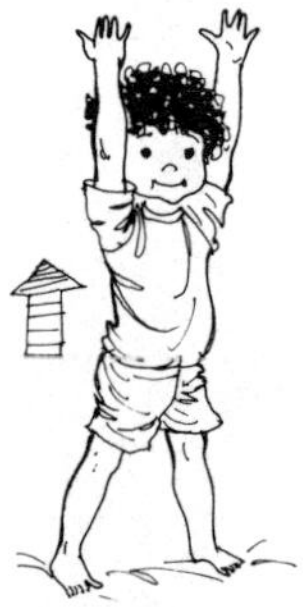

Count 1 - Flip Up

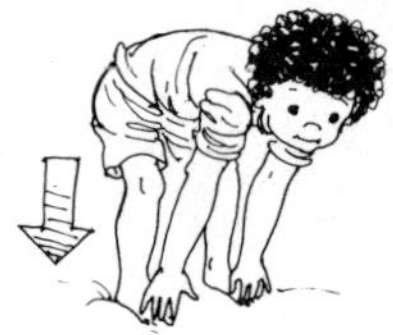

Count 2 - Flop

OPEN AND CLOSE THE GATE

Ready - Take stride position, elbows up, fingertips touching in front of chest.
Count 1 - Swing arms wide to sides, shoulder high.
Count 2 - Bend elbows, bringing arms back to ready position.

Repeat opening and closing gate several times.

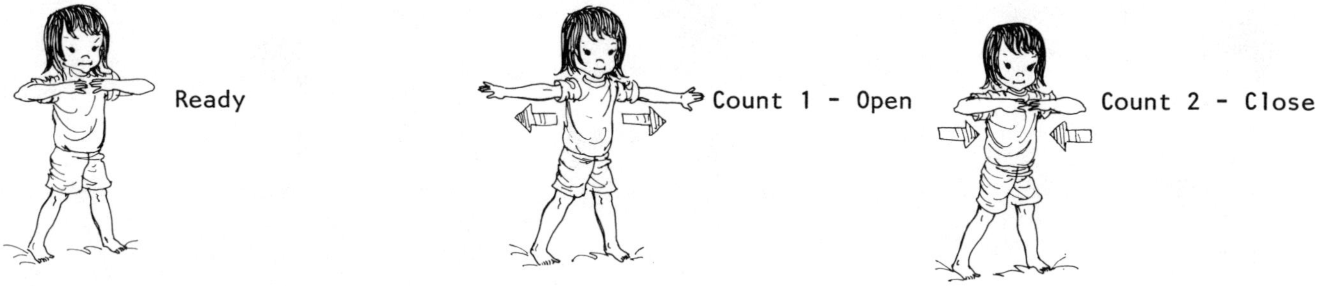

BIRDS FLY

Ready - Take stride position, arms hanging at sides.
Count 1 - Raise extended arms quickly sideward.
Count 2 - Lower arms vigorously, without slapping sides.

Repeat wings up and down several times.

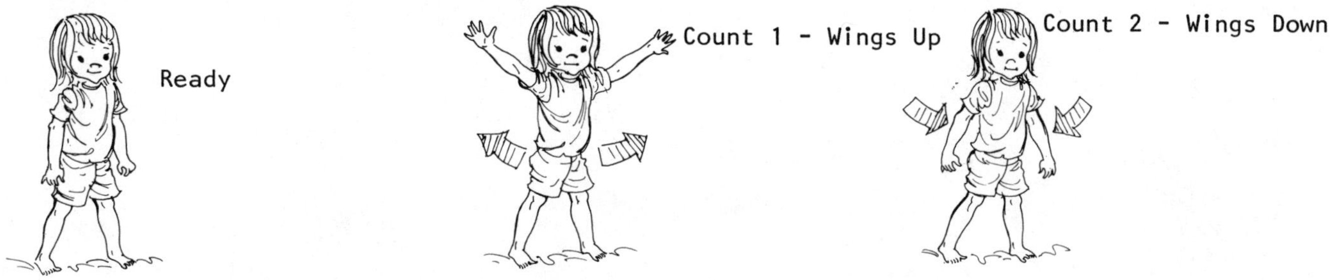

LEG DEVELOPMENT CHALLENGES

KANGAROO JUMP

Ready - Stand straight, arms bent in front of body.
Count 1 - Bend knees and waist slightly and jump forward, pushing off and landing with both feet, arms still bent.
Count 2 - Straighten body with head high, and look all around.

Repeat jumping and looking several times.

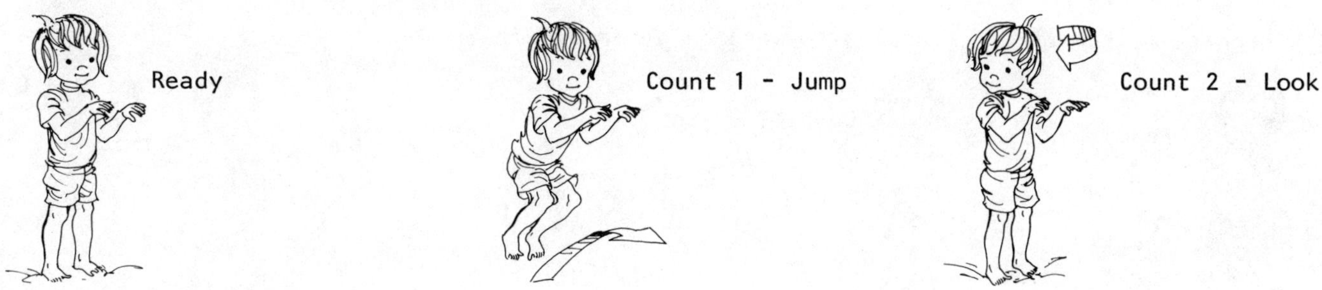

BOUNCING BALL

Ready - Stand straight, arms hanging at sides.
Count 1 - Bend knees and jump up, landing facing to the right.
Count 2 - Keep feet on the floor and do bouncing motion with knees.

Repeat big and little bounces, alternately facing to the right, then left.

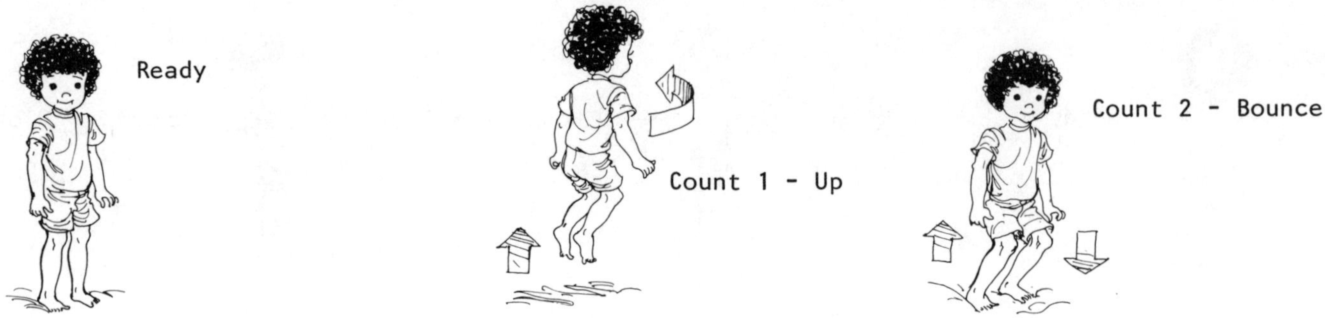

MR. JACK-IN-THE-BOX

Ready - Stand straight, arms hanging at sides.
Count 1 - Squat, feet slightly apart, arms crossed on chest.
Count 2 - Spring up to stride position, extending arms vigorously.

Repeat squatting and springing up several times.

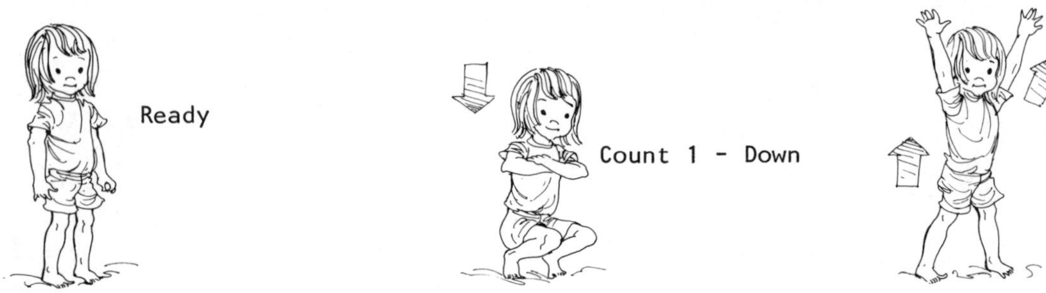

TRUNK DEVELOPMENT AND FLEXIBILITY CHALLENGES

BEAR HUG

Ready - Take stride position, arms hanging at sides.
Count 1 - Step forward with one foot, keeping other foot in place.
Count 2 - Bend at waist and hug extended leg with both arms.
Count 3 - Straighten up.

Repeat several times, stepping forward on alternate feet.

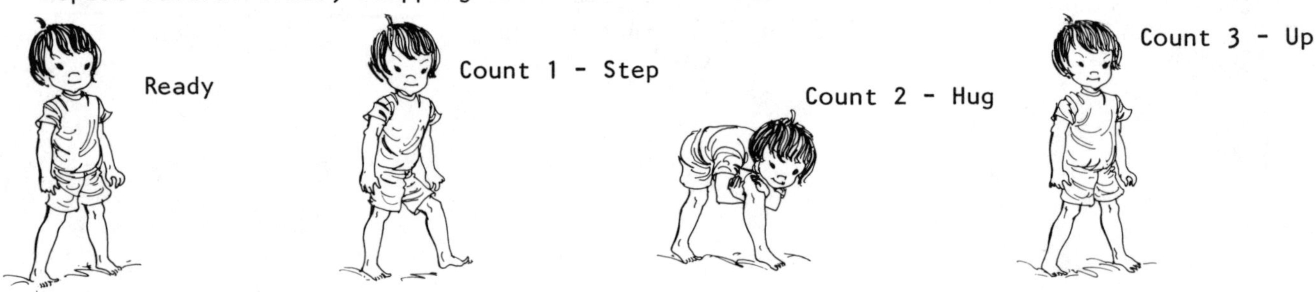

TREES IN THE WIND

Ready - Take stride position, arms overhead, hands relaxed.
Count 1 - Sway body and arms to right and straighten up.
Count 2 - Sway body and arms to left and straighten up.

Repeat several times, alternating swaying to right and left.

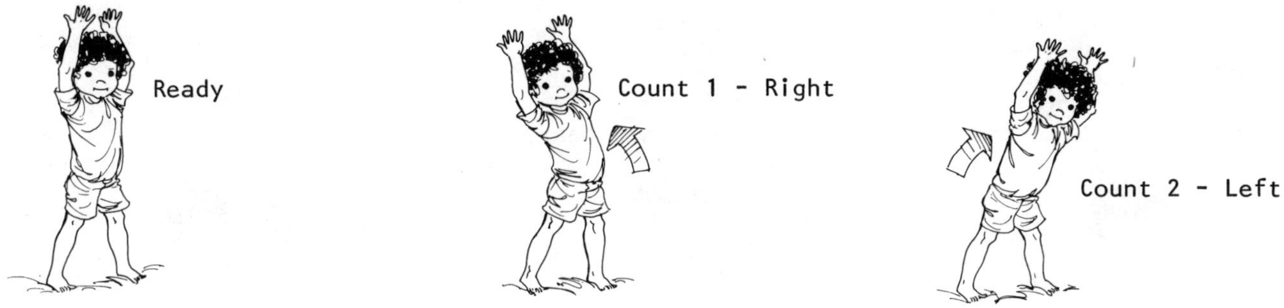

BUS STOPS
Ready - Stand straight, hands on hips.
Count 1 - Bend forward at waist, touching knees with fingers.
Count 2 - Bend farther, touching ankles with fingers.
Count 3 - Bend farther, touching floor with fingers.
Count 4 - Return to ready position, with hands on hips.

Repeat knees, ankles, floor, and up several times.

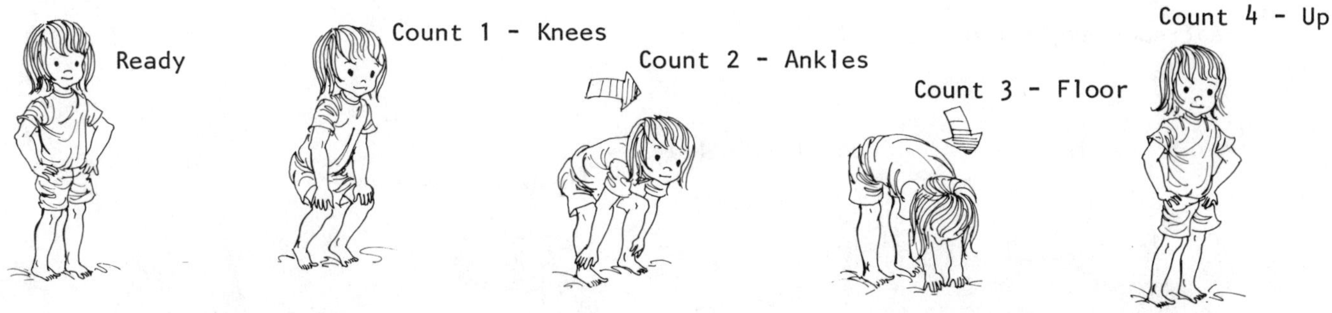

BALANCE AND COORDINATION CHALLENGES

TIGHTROPE WALKER
Ready - Stand straight, arms extended sideward, shoulder high.
Count 1 - Step forward (on painted line) touching heel of forward foot to toes of foot in back.
Count 2 - Step forward with other foot, placing it in like manner.

Continue walking without stepping off line or losing balance.

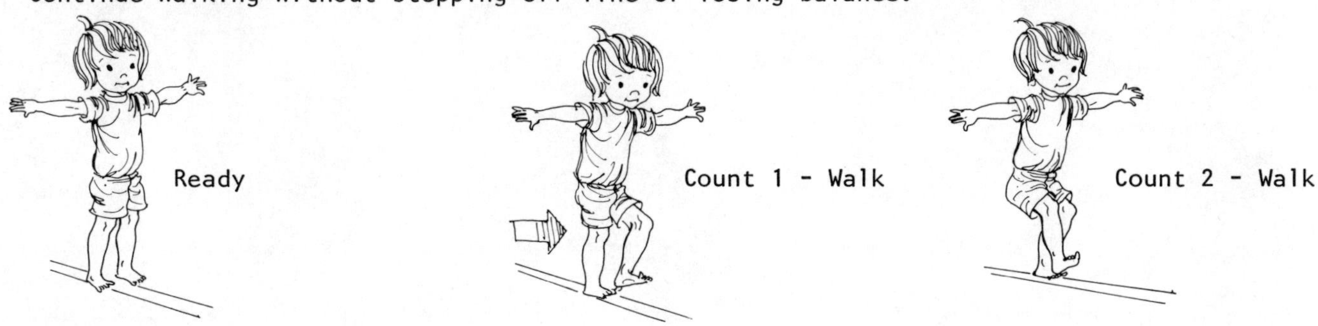

ANIMAL WALK
Ready - Take all-4's position, both hands and both feet on the floor.
Count 1 - Take a step forward with one arm and one leg.
Count 2 - Step forward with other arm and leg.

Continue walking on all-4's, like a dog, cat, bear, etc.

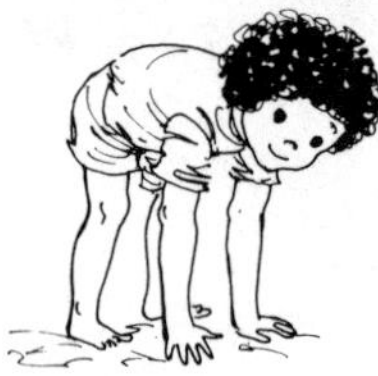
Ready

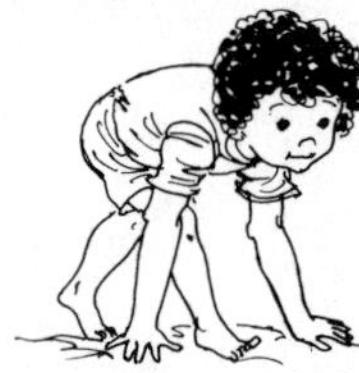
Count 1 - Step

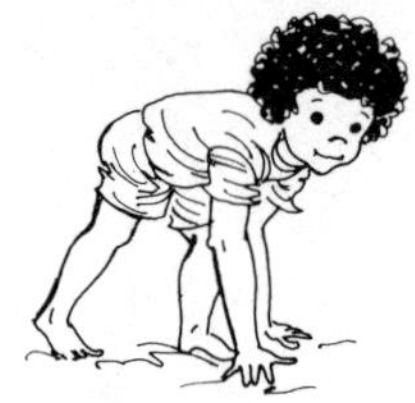
Count 2 - Step

JET TAKE-OFF

Ready - Take stride position, arms hanging at sides.
Count 1 - Squat down with fingers touching floor between knees.
Count 2 - Straighten knees, keeping fingers still on the floor.
Count 3 - Straighten body, flinging arms forcefully overhead, either rising on toes or giving an upward jump.

Repeat complete action several times.

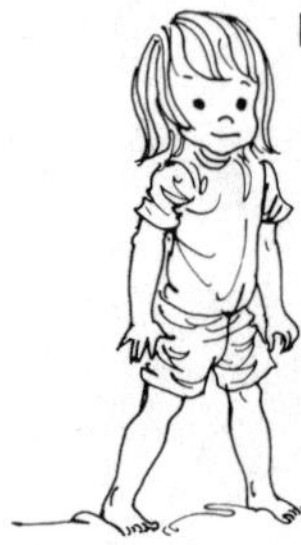
Ready

Count 1 - On Marks
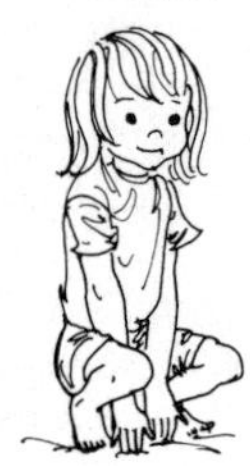

Count 2 - Get Set
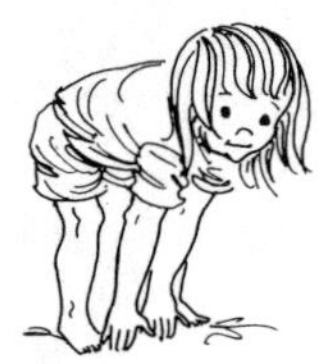

Count 3 - Blast Off!
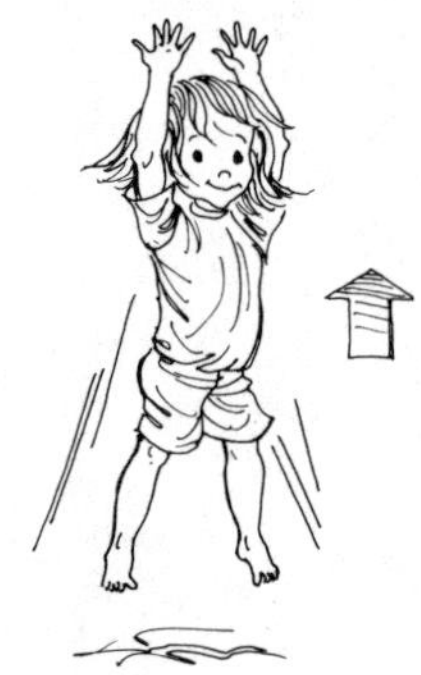

CIRCUIT TRAINING CHALLENGES

PERFORMANCE OBJECTIVES

By performing the following challenges, student demonstrates cardio-vascular endurance, strength, flexibility, agility, and gross motor coordination.

EQUIPMENT

This will vary according to the types of circuits planned. Circuits can be organized using no equipment or a wide variety of equipment.

GENERAL INFORMATION

Circuit training is a technique widely used in physical education programs to develop the above mentioned objectives. (Circuit training is especially useful in developing strength, endurance, and cardio-vascular fitness. Cardio-vascular fitness is related to the proper functioning of the heart and lungs.) The circuit principle, which uses a series of exercises to be completed in a timed interval, can be readily adapted to elementary physical education programs. It requires little or no apparatus and the circuits can be designed to utilize grass or asphalt play areas. The activities described in this section as well as many other calisthenics and self-testing activities, are used in circuit training.

No one questions the value of our need for daily vigorous activity. Elementary school teachers seek additional "vigorous activities". Circuit training, in contrast to routine formal exercises, provides interesting and exciting challenges for individuals to develop at their own speed.

Circuit training is an excellent method of body conditioning, not a program in itself. It should be used in conjunction with skill development, team games, and other activities in a well balanced program. The contribution it can make to physical fitness is so great that it could be well used once or twice each week.

Some will want to use a "Circuit" for the first 5 or 10 minutes of the period, followed by a game or a related activity. Others may want to use it for the entire period.

It is hoped that this brief description will provide enough information for creative teachers with imagination and a desire to make "fitness" a part of their physical education program, to find ways of including this activity in their program.

GROUP CIRCUIT TRAINING

Before starting a Circuit Training Program teach several exercises or activities such as the Jumping Jack, Push-Up, Wing Stretcher, Burpee, etc. Emphasize proper form, be sure the class becomes familiar with the exercises by name. This must be done before the Circuit Training principle can be introduced.

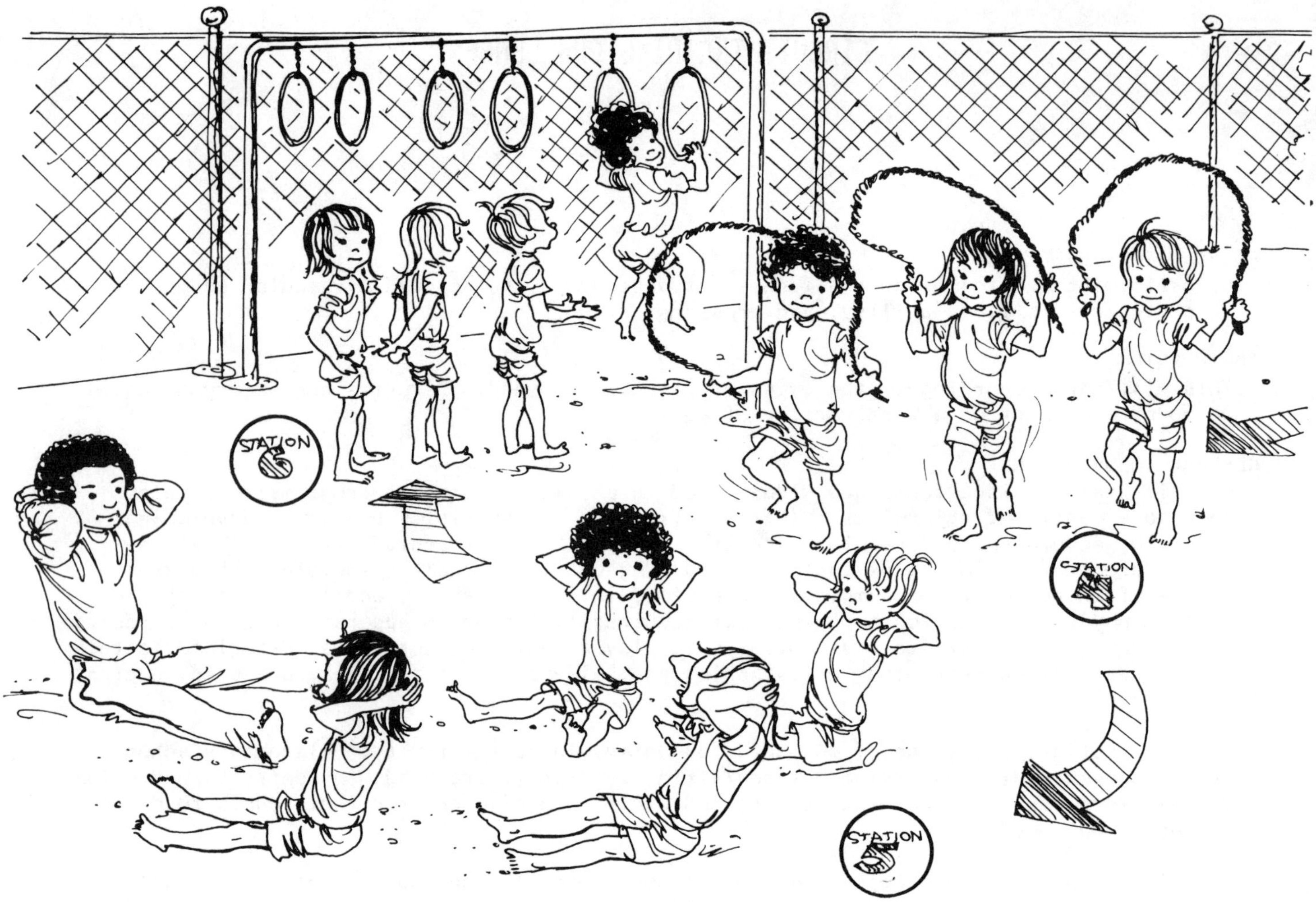

ORGANIZATION

The following organizational recommendations are illustrated in the 2-page drawing on this page and page 91.

1) Select a starting point on the playground, perhaps a painted circle or a large 4 square area. This is Station 1. The group can place themselves around the circle or square facing a leader in the center. At this station complete a series of perhaps 10 or the following: a) Jumping Jacks; b) Burpees; and c) Alternate Toe Touching.
2) Briskly walk to Station 2 (a previously designated area perhaps 25 to 50 yards away). At this station do a new series of activities such as: a) Wing Stretcher; and b) Push-Ups.
3) Jog (a slow run) to Station 3. At this station perform a Bear Walk (sideways on all 4's) about the length of an outdoor basketball court.
4) Run at 2/3rds speed to Station 4. At this station do a series of Rope Jumps (between 25 and 50 jumps). Have enough ropes present so that each member of the group has one rope to jump with.
5) Sprint at full speed to Station 5. At this station do a series of Sit-Ups. If done on asphalt, have mats present.

By this time in the Circuit the heart beat should be greatly increased. Circulation is more rapid, blood with a fresh supply of oxygen will be distributed throughout the body. The goal will be to continue this increased circulatory/respiratory action for a period of time. *Never stop moving.* The student is running, jogging, briskly walking, or doing

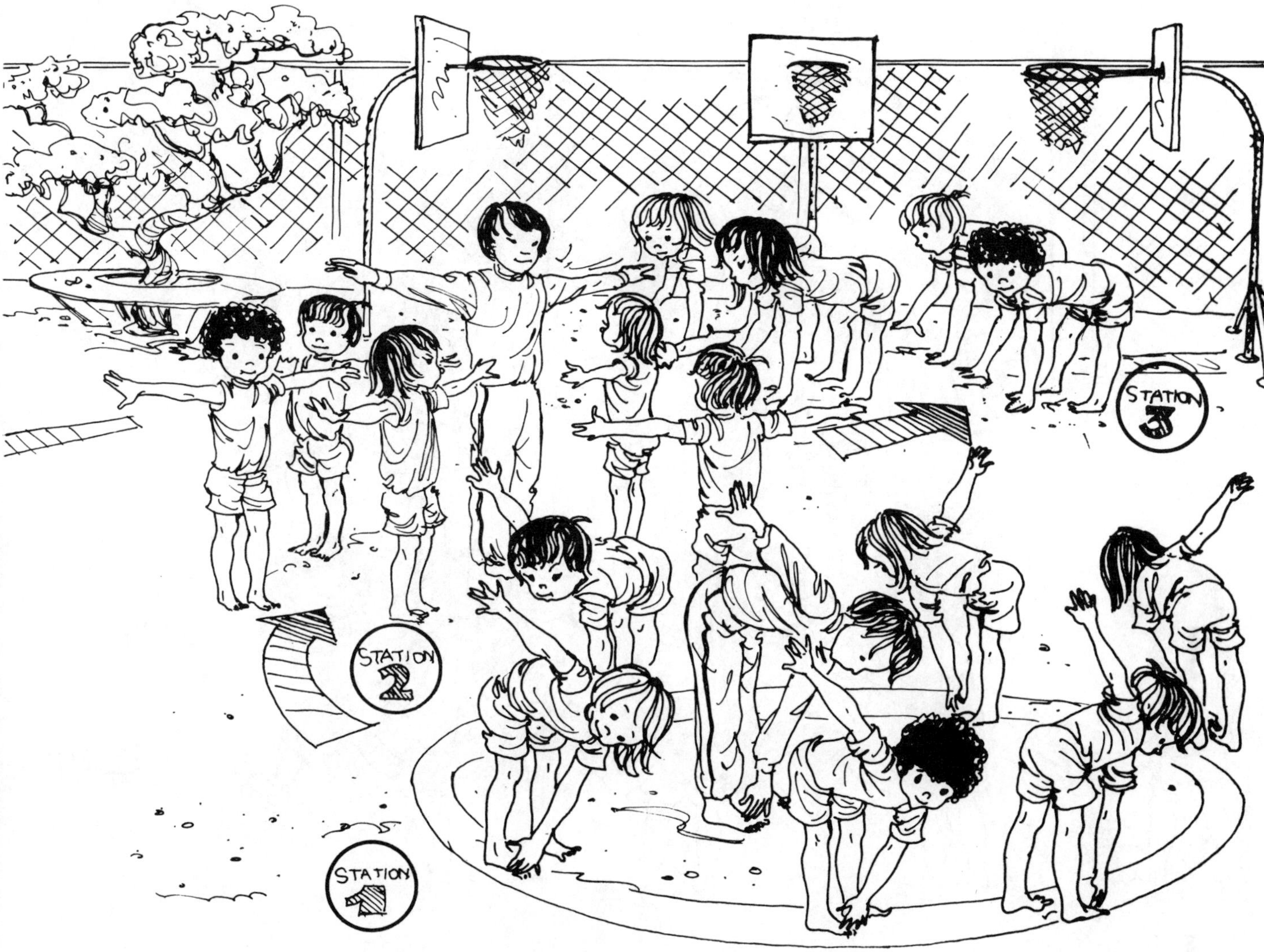

some activity all the time. Continuous action is a new sensation for many students. The natural impulse is to stop whenever the feeling of fatigue is experienced.

6) Run at 2/3rds speed to Station 6. Do a series of: a) Pull-Ups; b) Travel The Horizontal Ladder; c) Turn Over The Low Turning Bar; and d) Travel On The Monkey Rings.
7) Jog once or twice around the turf or asphalt area, depending on its size.
8) Briskly walk to the starting point or Station 1 and taper off with: a) Deep Breathing; b) The Swimmer (bend forward at the waist and do the crawl stroke in swimming); and c) Arm Rotators.

TEACHING SUGGESTIONS

1) Establish a "Target Time" for the entire class. The "Target Time" is the time it takes the class to complete the entire circuit. Each week, this time can be reduced as strength and endurance are developed.
2) Select 2 or 3 groups in the class, based on their time in completing the circuit. Group 2 starts the activities at Station 1 when Group 1 (having completed the activities at Station 1) arrives at Station 2. Now each group can establish its own "Target Time". An alternate plan would be to have Group 1 start the circuit from Station 1, Group 2 from Station 2, etc. Each group completes the circuit at the station from which they start the course.

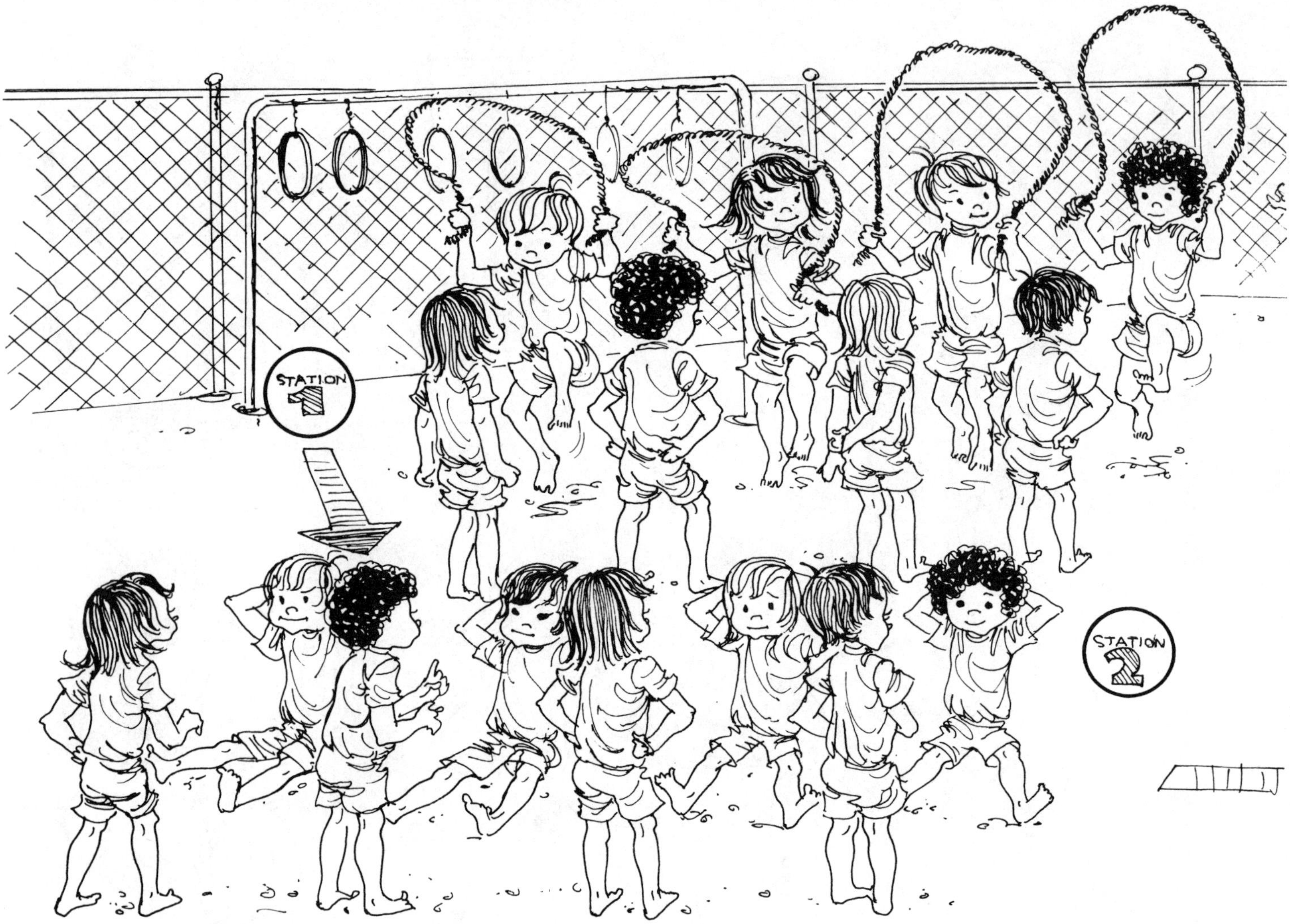

3) Establish definite locations for each station. Establish definite exercises and a definite number of times to do each exercise. As skill improves, increase the exercises and/or the number of times each activity is to be executed.
4) Require 2 or 3 trips around the circuit as skill increases.
5) If the playground is adequate, plan an interesting circuit that travels over the entire area. On more limited playgrounds, the stations can be adjusted back and forth across the field or asphalt area.
6) Use individual pieces of apparatus or the apparatus area as a station. Many activities using playground apparatus are excellent such as chinning, traveling the horizontal ladder, using the low turning bar, etc.
7) Emphasize the principle of continuous motion, never stop moving from the time the first exercise is started. Tapering off or recuperative activities should be done at the last station. Gradually return the heartbeat to normal.
8) Increase the amount of brisk walking, running, jogging, and sprinting. Require a lap of the field between each station instead of merely moving to the next station.
9) Build for character. Instill the idea of personal development, no cutting on the number of repetitions, no cutting on an activity, etc.
10) Increase the number of stations or decrease the number to fit your play area. Also, increase or decrease the variety of activities and the number of repetitions to fit the needs of your group. Stations may include sport skill activities for variety such as basket shooting, dribbling a ball around obstacles, volleying a ball against a wall, etc.

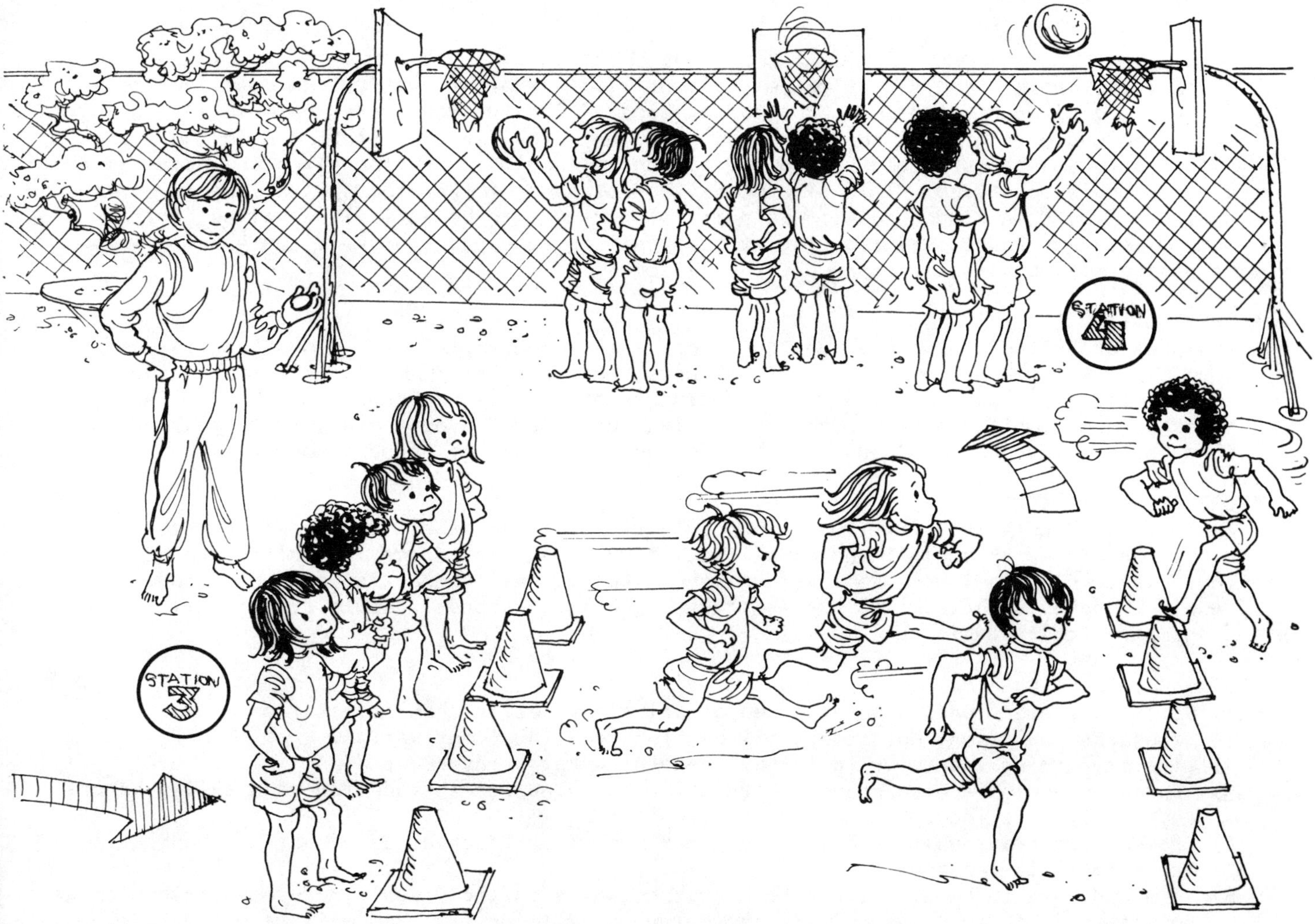

PARTNER CIRCUIT TRAINING

ORGANIZATION

The following organizational recommendations are illustrated in the 2-page drawing on pages 92 and 93.

A planned number of circuits (stations) are arranged within the available space. Usually 4 to 8 stations will be appropriate depending on class size. Each student is paired up with a partner (preferably of similar ability) and the same number (pairs) of partners are assigned to each station. The number of students at each station may vary slightly so long as each student has a partner and enough equipment is available. The instructor is positioned with a stop watch in the center of the circuits as shown in the above 2-page drawing. During each time trial half of the students will perform while the other half serve as counters and/or recorders. At the end of the first time trial, the partners change places and are ready for the 2nd time trial. At the conclusion of the 2nd trial, all students rotate to the next station in order of arrangement. The same process repeats with 2 new time trials. At the end of the lesson all students will have performed for a given time period at each of the planned stations. Scores may or may not be recorded depending on the desires of the instructor. Commands such as "Performers Ready", "Begin", "Stop", "Rotate Stations", etc., should be used to keep the lesson running smoothly. The entire lesson should be run in a well organized and "snappy" fashion.

The key factor in organizing timed circuit drills is that *all activities must lend themselves to a given time period (30 seconds, etc.)*. Careful consideration must also be given to the amount of equipment needed at each station. For example, Station 1 in the 2-page illustration on pages 92 and 93 shows 8 students (4 pairs of partners) which indicates that 4 ropes would be needed. This also means that at each of the other 3 stations shown, enough equipment would be needed to allow 4 pairs of partners to be actively involved at the same time. For basketball shooting at Station 4 on page 93, 4 baskets and 4 balls would be needed to successfully carry out the lesson.

FITNESS STATIONS

Examples of "Fitness Stations" you could use are: rope jumping, sit-ups, step test on wood blocks or bench, push-ups, squat thrusts, hoop or tire rolling, agility running around obstacles, lateral (sideward) jumping through tires or hoops, shuttle run through tires or hoops while passing bean bags, 4-legged run around obstacles, obstacle run through, over, under, and around obstacles, and hoop jumping through hoops.

SPORT SKILL STATIONS

Examples of "Sport Skill Stations" you could use are: basketball shooting; basketball dribbling around obstacles; basketball wall target passing; soccer dribbling around obstacles; volleyball wall volleys; volleying volley ball to partner over net; base running; hockey dribble using hockey sticks, pucks, and cones; paddle tennis ball tapping; and paddle tennis ball bouncing.

TEACHING SUGGESTIONS

1) Self-improvement should be stressed at all times rather than competition.
2) Standards may or may not be established for individual motivation.
3) Class recording sheets or individual recording cards may be used.
4) Students should receive proper instruction and practice in technique and skills before any activity is incorporated into a circuit.
5) Praise for individual improvement and maximum effort regardless of ability and performance level is important.
6) If awards are to be given, try to base the awards on individual improvement/achievement so that all students, especially those low in skill or fitness, will be motivated to improve.
7) Students are alternating periods of stress (performance) with periods of rest (counting/scoring) which keeps enthusiasm high.
8) These same types of circuits (stations) may be organized without the stress of time trials. Self-testing activities can be presented using many different approaches.
9) Circuits should be rotated throughout the school year for variety and continuous enthusiasm. However, if improvement is to be measured, some core (basic) stations such as sit-ups and rope jumping should be used with consistency.
10) Circuit training may be planned for an entire class period or for a portion of a period. This, of course, is controlled by the duration of time trials and the number of stations used.

OBSTACLE COURSE CHALLENGES

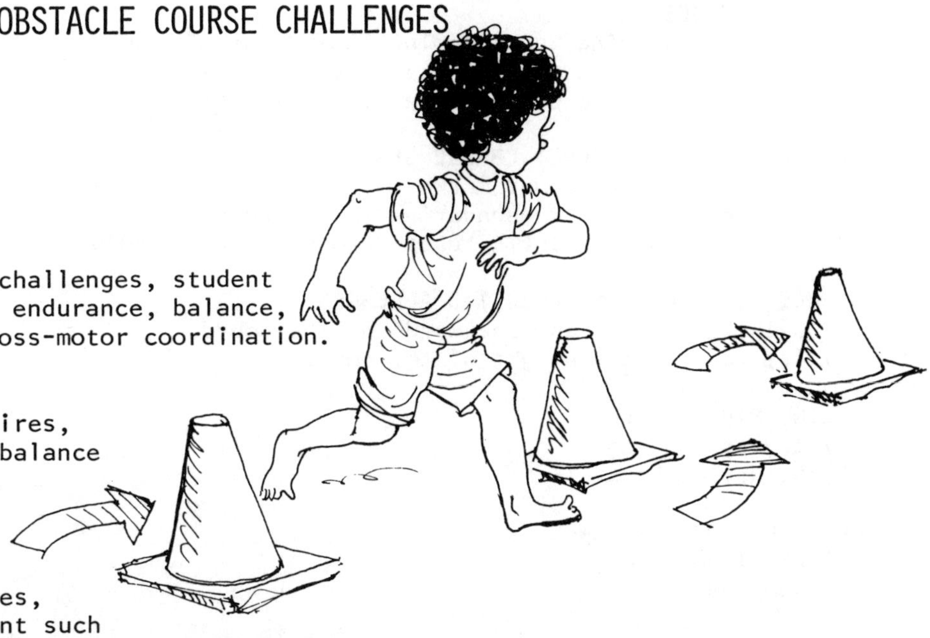

PERFORMANCE OBJECTIVES

By performing the following challenges, student demonstrates cardio-vascular endurance, balance, flexibility, agility, and gross-motor coordination.

EQUIPMENT

Jump ropes, tumbling mats, tires, traffic cones (game cones), balance beams, bowling pins (traffic cones can be used here too), cardboard boxes, large wood blocks, plastic bottle, wood benches, tetherball poles, hoops, and apparatus equipment such as low turning bar, horizontal bar, horizontal ladder, monkey rings, and climbing bars.

GENERAL INFORMATION

A motor-fitness challenge course involves a series of obstacles (stations) which are so arranged as to provide each student a variety of movement experiences. Each student relates to the obstacles from within his/her own physical make-up. There are no failures and, as the students begin to realize that they can use their bodies to accomplish all types of physical challenges, they naturally develop a more positive self-image. Improved balance, spatial orientation, laterality, directionality, and body management as well as general physical fitness are a direct result of such planned activity. The obstacles may be arranged around a turf area, on a hard top play area, in a multi-purpose room, around the perimeter of a classroom, or a combination of the above areas. It may also include your playground apparatus area. Below are listed many types of equipment which may be used as obstacles or stations in a challenge course.

JUMP ROPE CHALLENGES

1) Arrange in parallel formation on ground for jumping and hopping over and between.
2) Rope jumping station (circle on hard top). Each student must jump a given number of times.
3) Tie between chairs, etc., for jumping over and crawling under.
4) Use long jump ropes to mark off areas for animal stunts such as bear walk, crab walk, rabbit hop, etc.

TUMBLING MAT CHALLENGES

1) Sit-up station (each student must perform a given number of sit-ups).
2) Forward roll and log roll station.
3) Standing broad jump station.
4) Use for animal walks.
5) Use for safety under other equipment such as standards with cross bars for jumping, tires for jumping and crawling through, other obstacles for crawling under, etc.

TIRE CHALLENGES
1) Running, jumping, and hopping in and out of the tires (bike tires).
2) Crawling through the tires (car tires) when supported in upright position.
3) Jumping into the center of a tire (bike tire) from a given height.

TRAFFIC CONE (GAME CONE) CHALLENGES
1) Zigzag running around markers.
2) Marking corners or boundaries to go around.
3) Place ropes or plastic tubes across top of 2 markers for jumping over and crawling under.

BALANCE BEAM (WALKING BOARD) CHALLENGES
1) Walking forward and backwards on the board.
2) Try to vary the height of the board.

BOWLING PIN CHALLENGES
1) Zigzag running.
2) Corner markers.

CARDBOARD BOX CHALLENGES
1) Crawling through.
2) Jumping over.

LARGE WOOD BLOCK (Kindergarten Type) CHALLENGES
1) Stepping up and down a given number of times with rhythm.
2) Jumping over.
3) Zigzag running.

PLASTIC BOTTLE CHALLENGES
Plastic bottles made from liquid detergent or soft drink containers.
1) Zigzag run.
2) Marking corners.
3) Leaping over.
4) Stepping over on a balance board.

WOOD BENCH CHALLENGES
1) Crawling under.
2) Jumping over.
3) Balance walking.

TETHERBALL POLE CHALLENGES
1) Climbing.
2) Zigzag running.

HOOP CHALLENGES
1) Hopping and jumping through the hoops placed on the ground in patterns.
2) Running through hoops supported in upright positions.

APPARATUS EQUIPMENT

LOW TURNING BAR CHALLENGES
1) Hip circles.
2) Sloth hang and travel.

HORIZONTAL BAR CHALLENGES

1) Pull-ups.
2) Arm swinging and release.

HORIZONTAL LADDER CHALLENGES

1) Travel by hands on rungs.
2) Travel by hands on siderails.

MONKEY RING CHALLENGES

1) Swinging from ring to ring.

CLIMBING BAR CHALLENGES

Climbing bars can be circular, rectangular, etc.

1) Climbing.
2) Hand traveling.
3) Exploration.

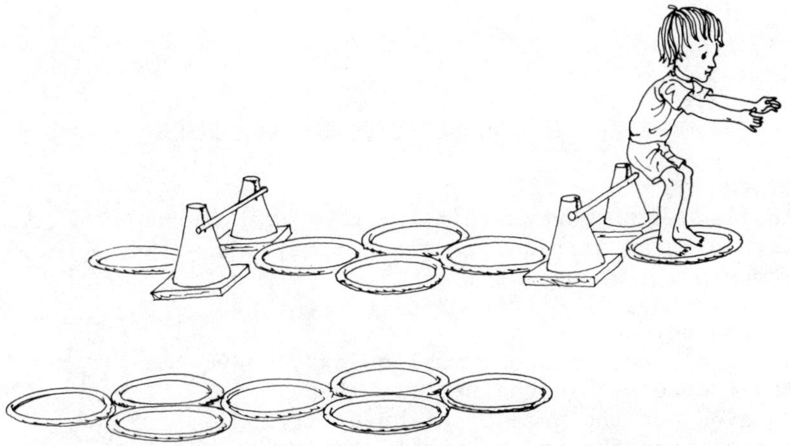

SHAPE AND NUMBER COURT CHALLENGES

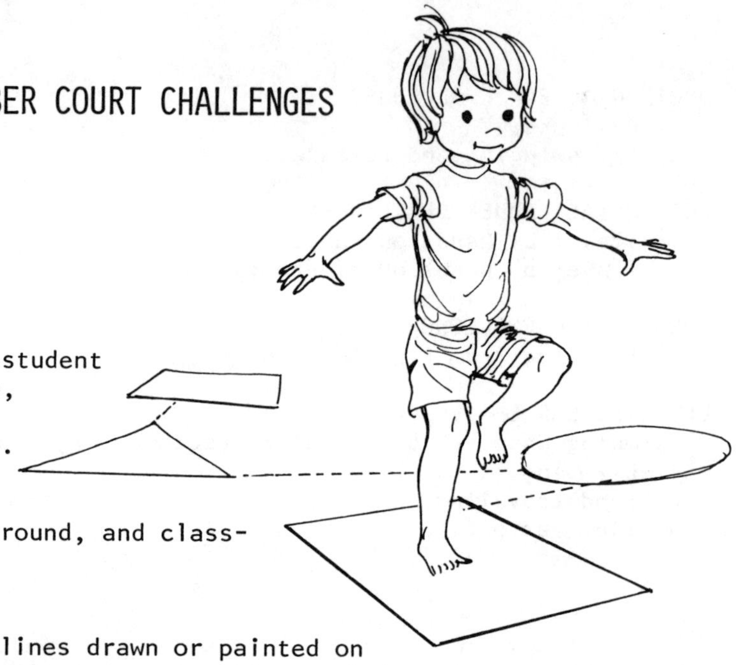

PERFORMANCE OBJECTIVES

By performing the following challenges, student demonstrates form and numbers perception, awareness of space, locomotor and ball skills, and recall and sequencing skills.

EQUIPMENT

Appropriate game courts painted on playground, and classroom set of balls.

GENERAL INFORMATION

Simple circles, squares, triangles, and lines drawn or painted on the playground provide teachers with excellent opportunities to help primary grade students develop and improve perceptual-motor skills. The activities suggested for each station only scratch the surface. For example, at the Shape And Number Circle station, you can easily work in addition and subtraction problems as well as a variety of kicking games. The painted game courts provide endless possibilities for motivating students to think, move, and learn.

SHAPE AND NUMBER CIRCLE CHALLENGES

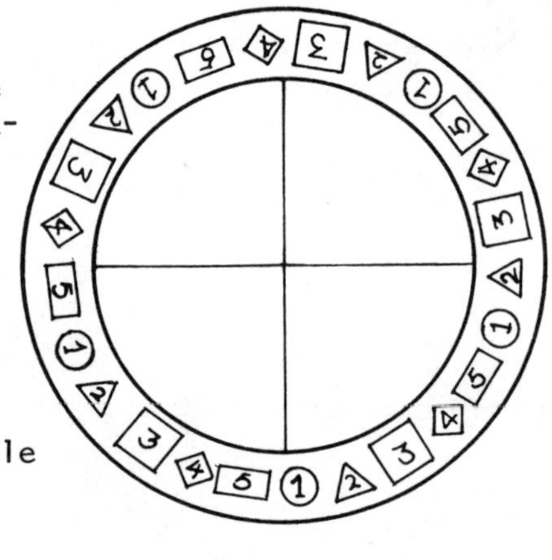

SPACE AWARENESS TRAINING

1) Students are challenged to move within the confines of the inner circle (see diagram at right). Teacher may use walking, running, hopping, jumping, etc.
2) Students continually move in different directions, but must avoid touching anyone.
3) On the whistle signal, each student must quickly leave the inner circle and freeze within the nearest shape.
4) As the teacher calls out the name of a shape (triangle, etc.), all students standing in the shape (triangle, etc.) resume movement within the inner circle.
5) Teacher calls out each of the shapes. Students must be able to correctly recognize the shape they are standing in.
6) Numbers may also be used along with the shapes.

LOCOMOTOR SKILLS

1) Students are challenged to move around the outside circle using the locomotor skill called by the teacher. (For example, skipping, sliding, galloping, running, etc.)
2) On the whistle signal, each student must freeze in the nearest shape.
3) Teacher calls out either the name of a shape or a number and students standing in that shape must raise their hands.
4) Instead of raising their hands, the teacher may ask students to hop or jump in place as many times as their number tells them to when their shape is called.

BALL SKILLS

1) Each student has a 6 inch or 7 inch rubber ball in their possession.
2) Students are challenged to move in various ways (hopping, jumping, etc.) around the circle carrying a ball, or they may be challenged to dribble the ball with their hands or their feet.
3) On the signal of a whistle they must freeze inside the nearest shape with the ball held in their hands.
4) As their shape is called out, they must toss and catch the ball as many times as their number tells them to, or the teacher may ask them to bounce and catch the ball, dribble the ball, etc.
5) Teacher may wish to have the students walk and dribble the ball inside the inner circle as their shape is called out. They must explore space and maintain control over the ball.

GAMES

1) *CIRCLE EXCHANGE TAG* - One student is "It" and stands in the center of the circle. Other students are each standing inside a shape, preferably only one student in each shape. When the teacher calls out a shape or number, all students in that shape must run through the inner circle and exchange places. If a player is tagged by "It" before getting inside a vacated shape, he or she becomes the new "It". Various locomotor skills may be used in place of running to add variety and skill to the game. Several times during the game, have all students rotate to a different shape.
2) *PIN THROW BALL* - Each student has a rubber ball in their possession and stands inside a shape. A bowling pin is set up in the center of the circle. One student is appointed pin guard and stands near the pin to protect it. When the teacher calls out a shape, all students standing in that shape may throw or roll their ball at the pin. If a student knocks the pin down, he or she becomes the new pin guard. The old pin guard takes his or her place in a shape. The thrown balls are immediately retrieved by those who threw the balls. (They retrieve a ball coming in their direction across the circle!) When the teacher says "Rotate", all the players should move to a different shape.
3) *STEAL THE BACON* - An eraser or bean bag is placed in the center of the circle. Each student stands in a shape (one student to a shape). The teacher calls out a shape and those students in the shape called attempt to retrieve the bacon and get it back to their shape without being tagged. One point is awarded for successfully retrieving the bacon. After each shape has been called at least once, the teacher should have the students rotate to a different shape.

NUMBER JUMP CHALLENGES

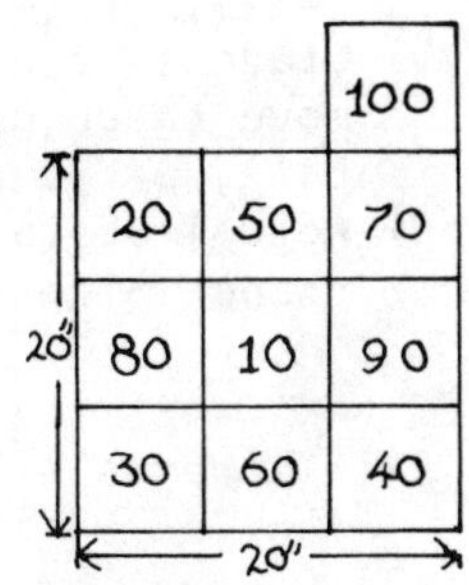

1) The jumper puts toes on the starting line (it may be any point outside the court) and takes off with both feet at once.
2) Student must land in square #10 and progress to square #20, then to square #30, and so on through to Square #100.
3) The jumper must make each jump without adjusting his or her feet. This means the player jumping must think one square ahead in order to land in the best possible position to make his or her next jump.
4) A player misses and must await his or her next turn if:
   a) Student moves his or her feet upon any landing.
   b) Student touches a court line.
   c) Student touches any part of his or her body other than feet to the ground.
5) The first player reaching square #100 would be the winner, or an optional method is to award one point to the player reaching the highest numbered square on each round of turns. In the optional method, the teacher can announce that the first player earning 5 or 10 points is the overall winner.

MOVEMENT PATTERN CHALLENGES

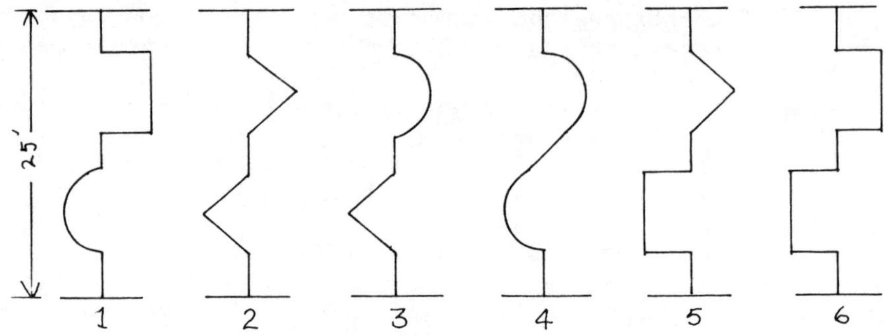

1) Students are divided up in even numbers ready to perform at each of the patterns.
2) Students are challenged to move through their patterns one at a time using various locomotor skills such as walking on tip toes, hopping, jumping, sliding, etc.
3) The object is to stay on the line of their pattern until they arrive at the end line.
4) After each student has had several turns to practice the skill at his or her assigned pattern, the groups are rotated to a new pattern.
5) The teacher now presents a new locomotor challenge. For example: Show me how you can skip the pattern; etc., and the activity continues.
6) Ball skills may also be incorporated by challenging the students to bounce and catch the ball while traveling on the line pattern, or by dribbling the ball, tossing and catching the ball, etc.

SHAPE AND NUMBER COURSE CHALLENGES

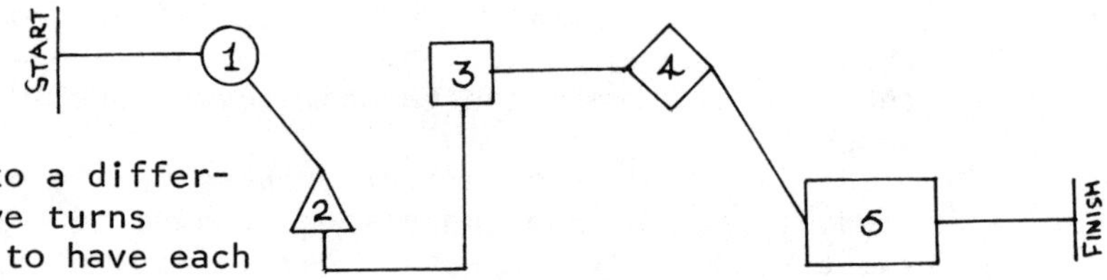

1) Teacher can lead the students in "follow the leader", moving through the challenge course using various locomotor skills. When arriving at each shape, the teacher can change to a different skill. Students should also have turns being the leader. Teacher may wish to have each student call off the name of the shape as the student reaches it.
2) Teacher can present movement challenge and shape recognition problem to individual students. Example, "Billy, can you hop on one foot to the triangle?" For greater challenge: "Ann, show me how you can gallop to the square and then skip to the rectangle."
3) Students can be challenged to move through the complete course using an assigned locomotor skill, or to create their own pattern of movement.
4) Students can be assigned to carry a rubber ball or jump rope as they are challenged to move through the course in various ways. At each shape they must bounce and catch the ball, or jump the rope, as many times as the number in the shape tells them to.
5) Actual obstacles (tires, jump standards, walking board, mats, etc.) can be placed on each shape which the students must react to as they move through the course.

APPARATUS CHALLENGES

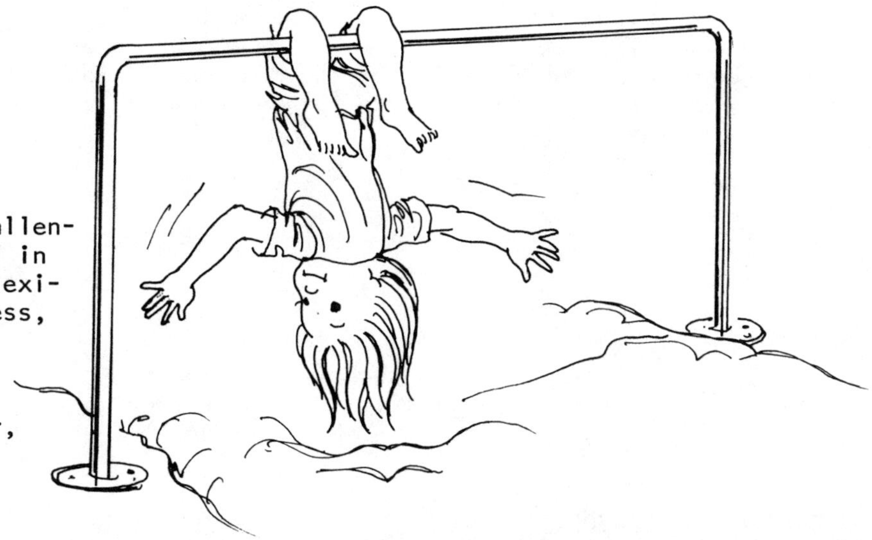

PERFORMANCE OBJECTIVES

By performing the following challenges, student demonstrates skill in body control and management, flexibility, strength, space awareness, and gross-motor coordination.

EQUIPMENT

Low turning bar, horizontal bar, jungle gym, horizontal ladder, and monkey rings.

GENERAL INFORMATION

Pre-school and elementary school children should have the opportunity of participating in *directed* and purposeful apparatus activity on a regular basis. This means that it is not just a recess activity or a free play period, but rather one in which *every* student is actively involved. The apparatus program should be structured by the teacher so that each student is exposed to certain basic body movement and control skills. Among the highly desirable outcomes of such planned experiences will be a greatly improved self-image and an increase in muscular strength especially in the vital upper trunk area. A fundamental need of all young, healthy, active students is to use their bodies to climb, hang, swing, jump, etc. These experiences were at one time a natural part of a growing child's environment. However, in today's society the schools must see to it that opportunities to meet these basic physical needs are provided.

GENERAL SAFETY PRECAUTIONS

1) Performers should use proper hand grips and always maintain a firm grip on the apparatus.
2) Apparatus should be used for activity, not as a resting place.
3) Performers should learn to land correctly.
    a) Bend knees immediately upon landing to absorb shock.
    b) Land lightly on balls of feet.
4) Each student should wait his or her turn at a safe distance from the apparatus.
5) Definite paths for entering and leaving the apparatus area should be used.
6) Do not allow pushing or grasping of performers by other students.

TEACHING SUGGESTIONS

1) First of all, explain the purpose and use of each piece of equipment to the students. Stress safety precautions!
2) Acquaint students with basic skills they will use or develop at each piece of equipment. Teacher will probably desire to use a student demonstrator and then allow each student to practice the activity.
3) After students are familiar with equipment, divide up into groups or squads and assign each squad a piece of apparatus.
4) Rotation between the various pieces of apparatus may be on a time basis (for example: every 5 minutes) or on completion of skill activity at each station.
5) Each week when the apparatus is used the teacher can position her or himself at a different piece of apparatus. This allows her the opportunity of working with each student at every piece of equipment.

TYPES OF APPARATUS GRIPS

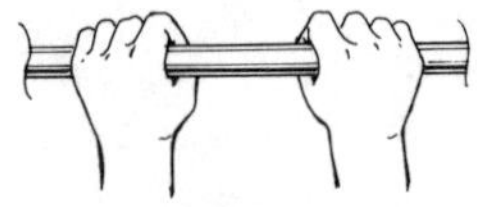

#1

1) *OVERHAND GRIP* - The thumbs are under the bar, fingers over it, and the back of the hands toward the performer.
2) *UNDERHAND (REVERSE) GRIP* - The thumbs are over the bar, fingers under it, and the palms of the hand toward the performer.
3) *MIXED GRIP* - Overhand grip for one hand and a reverse grip for the other.

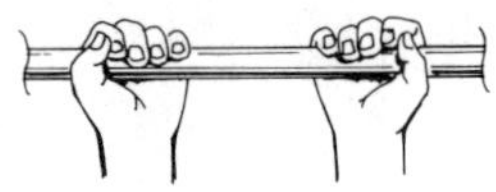

#2

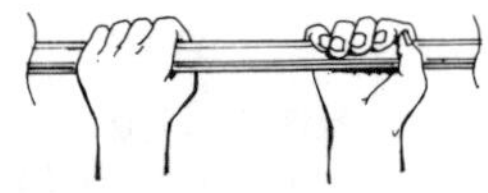

#3

LOW TURNING BAR CHALLENGES

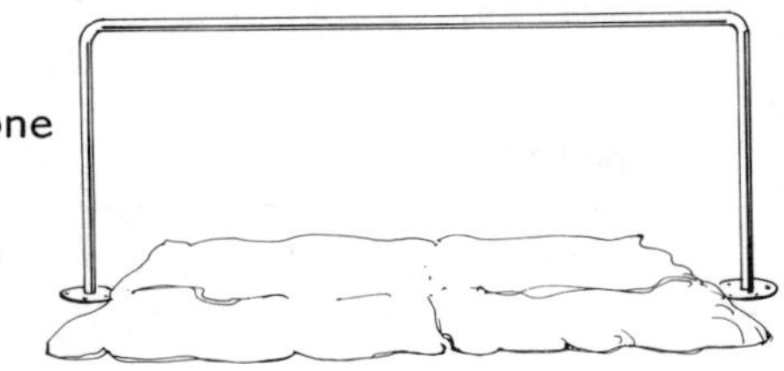

This piece of apparatus can usually accommodate 3 students at one time depending on the activity. Emphasize, for safety, that hands are *not* removed from the apparatus until feet are on the ground.

MODIFIED PULL-UP
1) Stand facing the bar, grasp with both hands, shoulder width apart, using overhand grip.
2) Walk 2 or 3 steps forward and lower body to hand position, weight supported by feet and hands. Keep body in a straight line from the heels to the shoulders.
3) Raise and lower body to bar by pulling up with arms, bending and extending arms as many times as possible. Keep body straight!

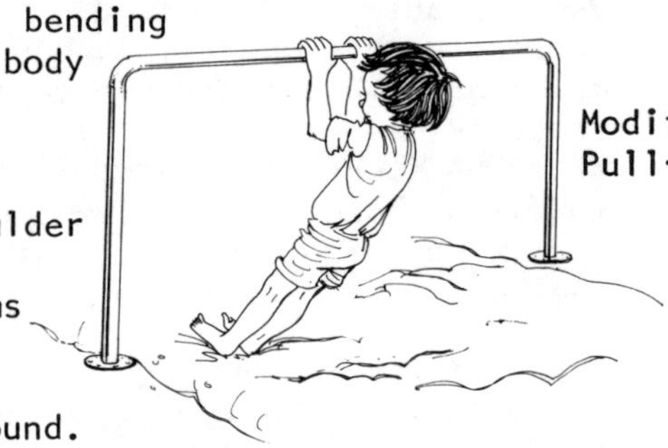

Modified Pull-Up

HIP CIRCLE (FLIP THE PANCAKE FORWARD)
1) Stand facing the bar, grasp it with both hands, shoulder width apart, using overhand grip.
2) Jump to a waist-leaning position on the bar with arms extended, change to underhand grip and turn forward, bending at hips.
3) Finish hanging by hands with feet resting on the ground.

Note that if the student cannot rotate forward, it is because he or she does not have enough weight above the bar.

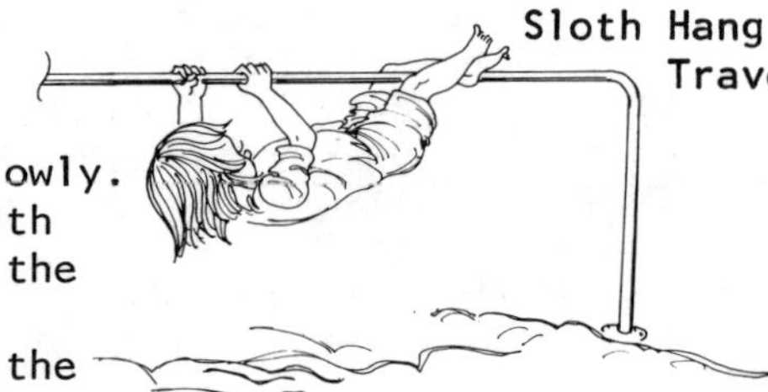

Sloth Hang And Travel

SLOTH HANG AND TRAVEL

A sloth is a South American animal that hangs from it's hands and feet on the branches of trees and moves very slowly.
1) Using an overhand grip, the performer grips the bar with both hands, but one hand comes over from each side of the bar.
2) Performer swings first one leg up on the bar and then the other. The legs should hook together at the ankles.
3) By moving the hands along the bar (pulling with the arms) and dragging the feet on the bar, the performer travels forward head first to the end of the bar.

KNEE HANG
1) Stand facing the bar, grasp the bar with one hand using an overhand grip.
2) Place the opposite leg over the bar, hooking the knee; grasp the bar with the other hand using an overhand grip.
3) Swing backward to an inverted position, hanging from both hands and one knee, now hook the other knee over the bar between the hands.

4) From an inverted hang position release one hand at a time until you are hanging from the knees only. To dismount, regrasp the bar with the hands and remove the legs from the bar.

SINGLE KNEE CIRCLE

1) Stand facing the bar, grasp the bar with one hand using an overhand grip.
2) Place the opposite leg over the bar hooking the knee, grasp the bar with the other hand using an overhand grip so that the knee is between the hands.
3) Mount the bar and change to an underhand grip, lock the foot of the hooked knee under the knee of the other leg, now turn forward.

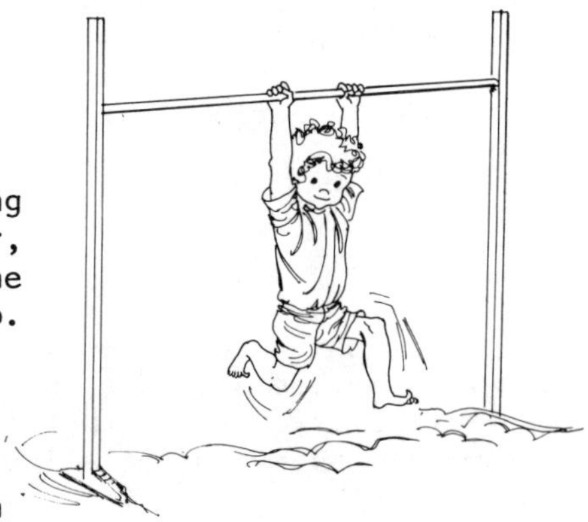

HORIZONTAL BAR CHALLENGES

One or 2 performers can be on the bar at the same time, depending on the activity. For safety, emphasize a locked grip on the bar, that is, if the fingers are over the bar, the thumbs go under the bar (overhand grip) and just the opposite for the underhand grip.

HANG AND DROP

1) Performer jumps up and grips the bar with both hands using the overhand grip.
2) The body should now be hanging in a fully extended position with the arms and legs straight. Feet are *not* touching the ground.
3) After hanging for several seconds, the performer releases the grip with both hands and drops to the ground.
4) Performer should bend knees and land lightly on the balls of the feet. Arms are out in front of the body for good balance.

HAND AND RIDE BICYCLE

1) Performer assumes the same positions as in the "Hang And Drop" challenge above.
2) Performer pumps legs with high knee action as if riding a bicycle. (This should not be a kicking action, but rather a pumping action.)
3) Challenge the student to see if he or she can do it for 5 counts, then 10 counts, etc.

HANG AND SWING

1) Performer assumes the same position as in the "Hang And Drop" challenge above.
2) Keeping body in an extended position, performer swings forward and backward.
3) After several trips forward and backward the student releases the grip and lands lightly on the balls of the feet.
4) Young students who are just learning this activity should not release the bar until the hips and legs are under the bar.

KNEE RAISE TO CHEST

1) Performer assumes extended arm hang position on the bar using an overhand grip. (Same starting position as above.)
2) Performer pulls up slightly on the arms, curls the body, and slowly brings knees up to the chest.
3) Performer slowly lowers knees down until fully extended body position is reached.

FLEXED-ARM HANG

1) Performer grips bar with both hands using an overhand grip.
2) Performer bends arms and pulls body up to a position where the chin is above the bar with the elbows fully bent. Legs are fully extended.

3) Performer locks grip and holds this position as long as possible. (For motivation the teacher may wish to time the student in seconds to see how long he or she can hold this position.)

Note that if student cannot pull him/herself up into the flexed-arm position, then the teacher should assist, or have a chair for the student to stand on. This is an excellent activity for development of upper arm strength.

PULL-UP

1) Performer assumes extended arm hang position on the bar using either an overhand or underhand grip.
2) Legs should be straight and feet are *not* touching the ground.
3) By pulling up with the arms the performer raises chin above the bar and then lowers the body down to the starting position.
4) The action in #3 above is repeated as many times as possible.

JUNGLE GYM CHALLENGES

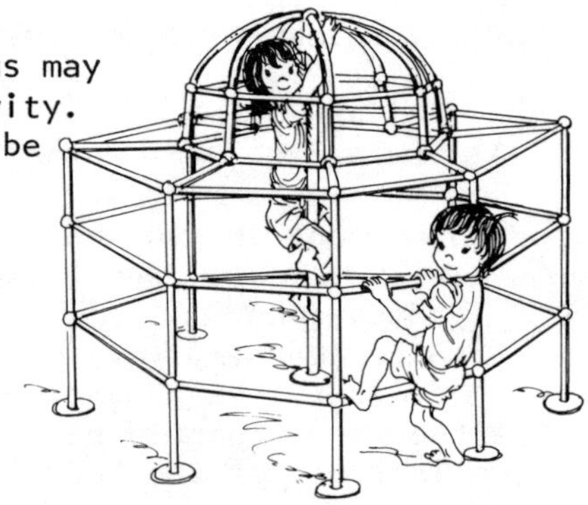

Sometimes shaped like a geometric dome, this piece of apparatus may accommodate 5 to 8 students at one time depending on the activity. For safety, stress that at least one hand and one foot should be on the apparatus at all times.

AROUND THE TOWN

1) Climb around the lowest level, keeping one hand and one foot on a bar at all times and gripping with the fingers over and the thumbs under the bars.
2) Return to starting place and leave the apparatus.

UP AND DOWN THE MOUNTAIN

1) Climb up and down the first 2 levels on the outside of the apparatus; moving alternately up on one section to the 2nd level and down on the next section to the first level.
2) Progress around the apparatus, return to the starting place, and leave the apparatus.

LOW ROUND TUNNEL

1) Climb around the squares of the lower level inside the apparatus.
2) Return to the starting place and leave the apparatus.

HIGH ROUND TUNNEL

1) Climb up one side, around the squares of the 2nd level, and back to the starting place.
2) Climb down and leave the apparatus.

FIREMAN'S SLIDE

1) Climb up on the outside to the 3rd level and slide down the center pole.
2) Keep hands on the pole and legs around it while sliding and exit at the opposite side.

HORIZONTAL LADDER CHALLENGES

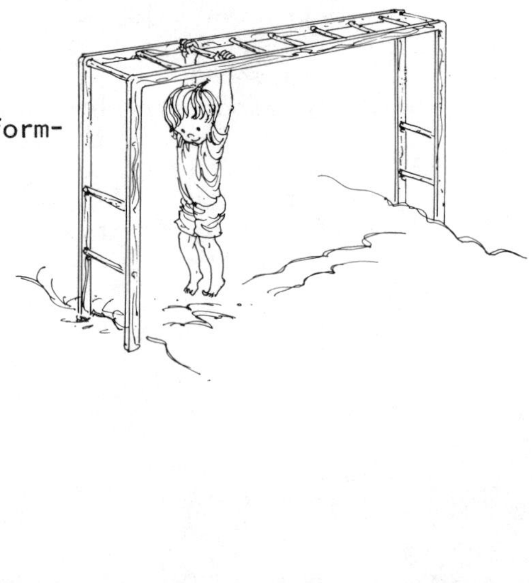

This piece of equipment may accommodate either one or 2 performers at the same time.

HAND AND DROP

1) Stand facing the end of the apparatus, place one hand on each supporting pole, climb both steps of the ladder.
2) Reach and grasp the 2nd rung of the horizontal ladder with one hand followed by the other, using overhand grips.
3) Hang for a moment and drop by looking at a landing place, letting go with both hands at once and landing lightly on the balls of the feet, bend knees immediately upon landing to absorb shock.

SWING AND DROP

1) Stand facing the end of the apparatus. Place one hand on each supporting pole and climb both steps of the ladder.
2) Grasp the 2nd rung with one hand and the 3rd rung with the other hand by using mixed grip. Palms are facing each other.
3) Facing the side of the ladder, swing the body from side to side.
4) Stop swinging, look at the landing place and drop by landing on the balls of the feet. Bend the knees immediately upon landing to absorb the shock.

SINGLE RAIL TRAVEL

1) Stand facing the end of the apparatus. Place one hand on each supporting pole and climb both steps of the ladder.
2) Grasp the first rung with both hands close together and near either side rail by using an overhand grip.
3) With the hand closer to the side of the ladder, reach and grasp nearer the side rail. Follow with the other hand by using overhand grips with palms of both hands facing in.
4) Travel sideways toward the end of the ladder as far as possible by sliding one hand and then the other.
5) Dismount by dropping or climbing down the ladder at the other end.

DOUBLE RAIL TRAVEL

1) Stand facing the end of the apparatus. Place each hand on a supporting pole and climb both steps of the ladder.
2) Grasp both side rails with the palms of both hands facing in and swing to a hang position.
3) Travel forward, as far as possible, sliding one hand and then the other.
4) Dismount by dropping or climbing down the ladder at the other end.

SINGLE RUNG TRAVEL

1) Stand facing the end of the apparatus. Place each hand on a supporting pole and climb both steps of the ladder.
2) Grasp the first rung of the horizontal ladder with both hands using an overhand grip and swing to a hang position.
3) Grasp the 2nd rung with one hand and then bring the other hand to the same rung. (Or alternate hands so that only one hand grasps each rung of the ladder.)
4) Travel forward in this way as far as possible.
5) Dismount by dropping or by climbing down the ladder at the other end.

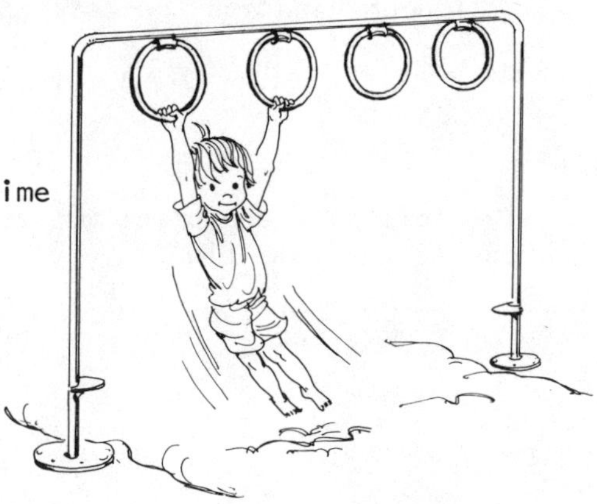

MONKEY RING CHALLENGES

One or 2 performers may be on this apparatus at the same time at the discretion of the teacher.

HANG AND SWING FORWARD

1) Performer grips one ring with both hands using an overhand grip. Body is hanging in fully extended position.
2) Performer swings forward and backward with a firm grip on the ring.

HANG AND SWING SIDEWARD

1) Performer grips one ring with the left hand and another ring with the right hand.
2) Performer swings in a sideward motion with a firm grip on each of the 2 rings.

SINGLE RING TRAVEL

1) Performer grips the first ring with both hands using an overhand grip.
2) Move one hand to the 2nd ring and begin to establish a swinging rhythm with the body.
3) Now, bring the other hand up to the 2nd ring or use an alternate ring method and bring this same hand to the 3rd ring.
4) Travel forward in this manner to the last ring and then drop or slide down the pole.

GAME CHALLENGES

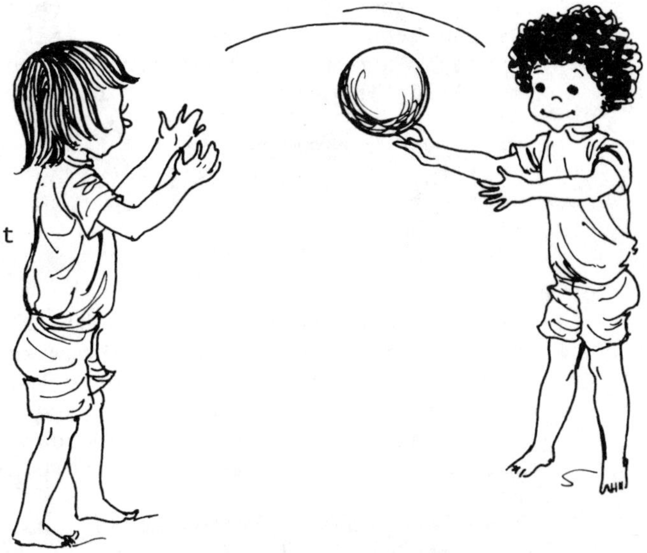

PERFORMANCE OBJECTIVES

By performing the following challenges, student demonstrates object handling skills, body and space awareness, locomotor skills, balance, and group cooperation.

EQUIPMENT

Equipment needs will vary depending on the game challenges selected for use. Many game challenges will not require any equipment.

GENERAL INFORMATION

Games can help to meet many important needs of children and, therefore, have an important role in the total physical education program offered. Unfortunately, games often become the total program offered in many elementary school programs. When this happens, children usually receive a "hit and miss" program with little planning and limited results.

Games recommended here are designed to enrich the total program and have been selected with basic needs of children in constant focus. These needs include vigorous activity such as running, the opportunity to develop physical skills such as throwing and catching a ball, learning concepts of sportsmanship and social interaction, leadership opportunities, developing listening skills, and the refinement of perceptual-motor abilities such as balance, body and space awareness, and directionality.

You will enjoy teaching these games and your students will have fun playing them as well as developing basic skills.

BASIC MOVEMENT GAME CHALLENGES

STATUES

1) The students form a straight line across one end of the playing area. One person is chosen to be the leader. He or she takes his or her place on a finish line, some distance in front of the group, with his or her back to the other players.
2) The leader counts aloud to a certain number, such as 10 or 15.
3) While the leader is counting, the players hop, run, or skip.
4) When the leader stops counting, the leader turns around immediately. At this time, all the players must remain motionless like statues.
5) Those caught moving must return to the starting line.
6) This is repeated several times.
7) The player who crosses the finish line first is the leader for the next game.

JUMP THE SHOT

1) Students form a large circle with one player in the center holding a rope. The rope is weighted at one end with a bean bag.

2) The center player starts whirling the rope with a steady motion close to the ground, so that the bean bag will reach the feet of the players in the circle.
3) As the bean bag swings around, each player jumps to avoid being hit.
4) A player who is hit must drop out until another player is hit. They then change places, resulting in only one player being out of the game at a time.

TEACHING SUGGESTIONS

1) This is a good skill game for eye-foot coordination.
2) Change the center player frequently.

DOUBLE CIRCLE

1) Students are arranged in a double circle.
2) Members of one circle face clockwise, members of the 2nd circle face counter-clockwise. Thus, the 2 circles will move in the opposite directions.
3) One circle has an additional player.
4) On a signal, the players skip around in their own circle until a whistle is blown or music is stopped, whereupon each player endeavors to secure a partner from the other circle.
5) The player who fails to secure a partner is said to be in the "mush pot".
6) Play is continued.

TEACHING SUGGESTIONS

1) Vary the game by having the players run, hop, or run on tiptoes, etc.
2) Do not permit boys to seek just boys, and girls to choose just girls unless the numbers are even.

JACK BE NIMBLE

For this activity use paper cones 6 to 8 inches high with a base not more than 6 to 8 inches across, representing candles, one for each group of players. (You may wish to try bowling pins, instead of cones.)

1) Students are divided into groups of 3 to 6 players.
2) Each group stands in file formation before its own candle.
3) On a signal, the first player in each file steps to his or her candle and jumps over it, jumping with both feet together.
4) Following the jump, on a 2nd signal, the player goes to the rear of his or her file.
5) Another signal is given for the 2nd player to jump, and so on, until each student has jumped over the candle.

TEACHING SUGGESTIONS

1) See that the students wait for commands and do not give the jumping signal until the previous jumper has reached the rear of his or her file.
2) Teach the students to use their arms for balance, and to land on both feet with the ankles, knees, and hips bent.

MOUSE TRAP

1) Students form a circle (the trap) by joining hands.
2) 5 students (the mice) stand outside of the circle.
3) To start the game, the teacher or leader calls "Open Trap." Students in the circle raise hands as high as their heads.
4) Leader calls, "Run little mice, run", and the mice (students outside the circle) run back and forth completely through the circle.
5) When the leader calls, "Snap" the students lower hands to waist level. (Do not let go of hands or stoop.)

6) Any mice inside of the circle are caught and join the circle or trap. Repeat until all mice are caught.
7) Choose new mice and start the game again.

TEACHING SUGGESTIONS

The number of mice may be changed according to the size of the group to allow more action.

SQUIRRELS IN THE TREES

1) 2/3rd's of the students form couples with their hands on the shoulders of their partners. In this manner they form hollow trees.
2) The trees should be scattered about in no set formation with considerable space between them.
3) The remaining 1/3rd of the students enter the trees as squirrels and stand there.
4) There should be one or more students without a tree home.
5) The teacher, or a leader, claps hands or blows a whistle, whereupon all the squirrels, including the homeless ones, run to secure a new home.
6) Squirrels who leave a tree may not return immediately to the same tree. The game is continued as long as desired.
7) 3 changes should be made in the positions of the players so that all the students have the chance during some part of the game to be squirrels.

TEACHING SUGGESTIONS

1) When the game is new, use only one homeless squirrel.
2) Do not permit 2 squirrels to occupy one tree.
3) Give the signals in rapid succession.
4) Have the trees scattered over an area large enough to encourage a vigorous run when the changes are made.

ONE-TWO-THREE

1) Class should be divided into 4 equal groups with each group assigned to line up on one side of a rectangular court area. (One group is on each side of the court to begin play.)
2) When the teacher blows the whistle *once*, all the students standing on the end lines move to the opposite end line. (They exchange places.)
3) When the teacher blows the whistle *twice*, all students standing on the side lines move to the opposite side line. (Exchange places.)
4) When the teacher blows the whistle *three* times, all students change to the *opposite* line.
5) Before blowing the whistle, the teacher should challenge the students to move with a definite locomotor skill (running, jumping, skipping, etc.).
6) Any students who a) move when it is *not* their whistle signal; b) use the wrong movement skill; c) collide with another student; are eliminated and line up at a designated spot.
7) Usually it is best to keep them out of the game for only a short period of time. A good rule is to allow one player to return to his or her side once another player has been eliminated.

TEACHING SUGGESTIONS

1) Multi-purpose game courts painted on playgrounds make a good game area.
2) This is an excellent game for developing listening skills, locomotor skills, and space awareness.
3) Use a wide variety of movement skills.
4) Ball skills may be worked into this game with each student having a ball in his or her possession.

SHIPWRECK

1) All participants are designated as members of the "Ship's Crew" and take a scatter position within the designated playing area. Playing area may be a multi-purpose room, turf area, basketball court, etc. They imagine they are on the deck of a ship.
2) Various commands (verbal challenges) are given by the teacher or leader. Participants must think and quickly respond.
   a) "Line up in the galley!" - Players quickly form a straight line down the center of the playing area.
   b) "Man the lifeboats!" - Players run to the left side wall, or left side boundary line.
   c) "Man the quarterdeck!" - Players run to right side of wall or right side boundary line.
   d) "Hit the deck!" - Players quickly lay down on the floor or ground. Depending on the type of playing surface, teachers may wish to modify the response to squatting down low.
   e) "Man overboard!" - Players assume a position on their backs with their feet and hands in the air. This command may also be modified, if necessary, to players taking a crab walk position (weight on hands and feet with stomach facing up).
   f) "Freeze!" - Players stop in place and hold position with no movement. This command can be given anytime the players are moving in one direction or another.
3) Challenges (commands) are given rapidly so that players must think and react quickly.

TEACHING SUGGESTIONS

1) Stress to players that they must think before they move.
2) Commands can be given in any sequence desired. Occasionally the same command may be repeated twice in succession to keep players alert.

WHISTLE MIXER

1) Students are scattered throughout the playing area (any large game court or designated area).
2) To begin the game, participants walk around in any direction they wish, but cannot touch. (They may also be challenged to skip, run, hop, jump, move fast, slow, high, low, etc.)
3) The teacher blows the whistle a specific number of times in succession with short, sharp blasts.
4) The students must respond according to the number of whistle blasts and form small circles with the number of participants forming the circle equal to the number of times the whistle is blown. (Example: If the whistle is blown 4 times, the students form a circle of 4 players--no more, no less.)
5) Any students left out (not forming in a circle) are eliminated. Also, if a circle is formed with more than the specified number of students, the entire circle is eliminated.
6) Eliminated students become game judges or officials on the sideline of the playing area.
7) The teacher now gives a new movement challenge and the game continues with students moving individually in different directions.
8) The game can continue until just 2 players are left who are declared the winners.

TEACHING SUGGESTIONS

1) If played inside (multi-purpose room) music can be added to make the game more enjoyable.
2) A good variation is to modify the elimination rule so that students are only eliminated for one turn. This keeps most players active at all times.

TELEPHONE POLES

1) Students are in scatter formation ready to begin play.
2) Teacher or leader calls out verbal challenges to students such as: "Who can balance on one foot?; Can you make yourself very small?; Try jumping like a kangaroo.; Shake your-

self out like a dust mop!; etc." Students use their imagination and respond to each challenge.

3) Whenever the leader calls out "Telephone Poles", all participants must react quickly and stand straight and still with hands at their sides like telephone poles.
4) Teacher may wish to keep students alert by attempting to trick them occasionally by calling out "Television", or "Telegraph Wires", etc., in place of "Telephone Poles".

TEACHING SUGGESTIONS

For variety and space awareness training use challenges such as: "Who can move about the available space like a tiger?;Show me how you can gallop like a horse?; Can you skip in a zigzag line?; etc."

TAG GAME CHALLENGES

ALL THE HORSES RUN

1) Players line up behind one of the 2 end lines.
2) The caller is in the center midway between the 2 lines.
3) The caller calls one person from the line. This person attempts to run to the other end line without being tagged by the caller. If this person is tagged, he or she joins the caller in the center.
4) If this person succeeds in crossing the other end line, he or she calls "all the horses run" and everyone starts running across the field.
5) The caller ("It") attempts to tag these people. The number of people called is generally equal to the number of people in the center (or one less, if you prefer).
6) The caller is the only person to call, and he or she may also call "all the horses run", and then everyone attempts to run.
7) The last one caught is the new caller. This is a tremendous physical fitness game with emphasis on endurance because of all the running involved.

TEACHING SUGGESTIONS

1) Emphasize that *all* taggers must be at midline before anyone is called to run. No runners run until all names have been called out.
2) Try variations such as: Caller can call out,"All boy horses run", or "All girl horses run", and Caller can use clothing colors in calling out groups of runners.

LEMONADE

1) The players are divided into 2 groups. A goal line is marked across each end of the play area and one group stands behind each goal.
2) The first group decides upon a "trade". They leave their goal and go to the opposite end of the play area, calling "Here we come!"
3) The 2nd group asks: "Where from?" First group answers: "New Orleans." 2nd group asks: "What's your trade?" First group answers: "Lemonade." 2nd group commands: "Show us some, if you're not afraid!"
4) Then the first group pantomines its' trade while the 2nd group tries to guess the trade. If the players guess correctly, they immediately give chase while the others run for their goal.
5) Any players who are tagged before reaching their goal become members of the side tagging them.
6) This game is repeated with the 2nd group choosing a trade.
7) The group of players who are guessing must maintain contact with its goal line until the chase begins.

TEACHING SUGGESTIONS

1) If the players need help in selecting trades, suggest such trades as washing dishes, making a cake, sweeping the floor, laying bricks, fishing, sawing wood, etc.
2) Keep the players in both groups spread across the width of the play area to avoid collisions as the players start to run.

CRACKERS AND CRUMBS

1) 2 teams of equal number are selected with one team designated the "Crackers" and the other team the "Crumbs".
2) Each team has its own safety (goal) line and there is also a center line from where the game starts. Each team lines up on the opposite sides of the center line, facing each other. Players should be encouraged to come close to the center line.
3) The teacher (or leader) will call out either "Crackers" or "Crumbs". The team called will turn and run back toward their safety line with the other team chasing them.
4) Any player tagged (touched) by the chasers must join that team. Both teams go back to the center line where the game continues with the leader again calling out either "Crackers" or "Crumbs".
5) At the conclusion of the playing time, the team with the most members is declared the winner. There is, however, no need to declare a winner.
6) The leader should make the game exciting and cause participants to listen carefully by calling out other "cr" sounding words such as, crazy, crows, critter, etc. Pointing one way and calling the other way will also keep the students alert.

FLOWERS AND THE WIND

1) The 2 groups, the flowers and the wind, are lined up on their own goal lines about 20 feet apart.
2) Teach the names of a few flowers.
3) The flowers secretly choose the name of a flower, then move up to face the wind.
4) The wind tries to guess the name of the flower selected.
5) When the right flower is called, the flowers turn and run for their own goal line chased by the wind.
6) Anyone caught by the wind must return with that group.
7) Have the groups alternate, one group being flowers, until all members of that group have been caught.

TEACHING SUGGESTIONS

Other subjects can be used, such as animals, birds, etc.

CIRCLE EXCHANGE TAG

1) Students form a circle and each student is given a number.
2) One student is then selected as the tagger and stands in the center of the circle.
3) The teacher or leader calls out numbers of the 2 students who must try to exchange places in the circle before the tagger can tag them.
4) Any player tagged becomes the new tagger and the game continues.
5) If the tagger does not tag either number called before they exchange places, then the tagger remains the tagger and 2 more numbers are called. (The teacher should know the number of the tagger so that it is not called out!)

PIRATE'S GOLD

1) Half of the group are "Pirates" and half are "Coast Guard".
2) Boundaries are set up with one goal line designated as "port" and another area (possibly a circle) as a "cave".

3) Pirates stand closely together in a cave and pass gold (bean bag or coin) to one of the players, keeping the Coast Guard (opposite team) from knowing which one has the gold.
4) Coast Guard players must stay in port (behind the goal line) until the captain of the Pirates calls out "Scatter!" This signals Pirates to scatter around the field (being decoys for the Pirate with the gold so that he or she can make "port") and for the Coast Guard to begin searching for the Pirate with the gold. (The gold cannot be transferred to another player after the Pirates leave their cave area.)
5) If a Pirate is tagged, he or she is told: "Hand over the gold." If he or she has the gold, he or she must show it and the Coast Guard wins the game (or a point). If the Pirate with the gold gets safely to Port, the Pirates win the game.
6) Game is then repeated with the Pirates being the Coast Guard and the Coast Guard becoming the Pirates.

HUNTER AND RABBIT

1) 2 people are "It" and each has a ball. The rest of the class line up on one end line. The 2 who are "It" are the hunters, while everyone else is a rabbit.
2) The hunters agree on a "movement" for the rabbits and call out: "Hop on one foot", "run", "walk", "jump", or any other call which all the rabbits must do.
3) The hunters must also perform the action and at the same time attempt to touch the rabbits with the ball or hit them with the ball by throwing it before the rabbits make it safely to the opposite end line.
4) The rabbits that are hit must remain where they are hit and are "poison" to touch any other rabbit who comes near them, who is then also caught. (The poison rabbits must not move from where they were hit or touched and use their hands to tag other rabbits within reaching distance.)
5) The last 2 rabbits caught then become hunters for a new game.
6) If a person (a rabbit) refuses to leave the safe lines at the end of the playing area, they (the hunters) may count 5, then tag that person anyway.
7) Anyone running outside the side boundary lines is caught.
8) Hunters must have a ball to tag a rabbit, which means that if a hunter throws a ball at a rabbit, he must retrieve the ball before he can tag another rabbit.
9) Each time the rabbits make it safely to the opposite end line, a new call (action) is made by the 2 hunters.

STEAL THE BACON

1) 2 equal teams line up.
2) A blackboard eraser or other object is placed in the center of the playing space between the 2 lines.
3) Each player has a number.
4) The leader calls a number and the 2 players holding that number go after the object.
5) The player that is not successful in getting the object, chases his or her opponent back, trying to tag the opponent.
6) One point is scored for each player returning to his or her line with the object without being tagged. (The end lines should be 20 to 30 feet apart.)

BALL HANDLING GAME CHALLENGES

TEACHER'S CHOICE

1) Players, about 4 to 8, stand on a line or in a line facing a classmate who is designated the teacher.
2) Teacher chooses the ball he or she wishes to use and throws it to each student in turn. (Equipment consists of different type and size balls for each playing group.)

3) Each player attempts to make accurate throws and good catches, using correct form.
4) When each student has received the ball, "teacher" goes to the end of the line and player at the head of the line (right side) becomes the new "teacher" and chooses a ball to be used.
5) Game continues until each player has been the "teacher".

TEACHING SUGGESTIONS

This is a simple type game drill to practice basic throwing and catching skills. Emphasize correct movement in throwing and relaxed catching action.

CIRCLE CALL BALL

1) Usually 6 to 8 players in a circle.
2) One person stands inside the circle and tosses the ball into the air while at the same time calling out the name or number of the players.
3) The person called on must catch the ball before it touches the floor.
4) If he or she succeeds, he or she becomes the leader and goes to the center. If he or she fails, the original center throws again.

TEACHING SUGGESTIONS

The vertical toss, as used in the game, is difficult for primary students. Often they throw the ball over their heads rather than throwing it vertically. The teacher can help them with this type of throwing by suggesting that they release the ball as soon as they have lifted it to a position directly in front of the chest rather than waiting until they have it at shoulder height.

CIRCLE-PIN THROW BALL

1) A 10 pin or bowling pin is placed in the center of a circle.
2) One person is selected to be the pin guard and tries to protect the pin from being knocked over by either one or 2 balls which are being thrown at the pin by class members lined up around the outside of the circle.
3) Any person who knocks the pin down becomes the new guard.

TEACHING SUGGESTIONS

Best to use either rubber balls or volleyballs. Teacher may wish to divide the class into 2 groups and have 2 games going at once. Good game for developing throwing for accuracy.

PIN BOUNDARY BALL

1) Players are divided into 2 teams.
2) Players of each team occupy the area between their own end zone and the center court line dividing the common rectangular playing field.
3) Each team has one ball in its possession (rubber ball or volleyball) and 3 pins located in its end zone. May use 2 pins per team instead of 3.
4) At a signal, members of each team attempt to throw their ball so that it will bounce, or roll across the opponent's end zone area and also possibly knock down a pin in the opponent's end zone.
5) One point is scored each time a ball rolls or bounces over a goal line.
6) 2 points are scored each time a pin is knocked down. (The pin stays down.)
7) Balls going across the opponent's end zone area on the fly *do not* score a point.
8) If a ball goes out of bounds before going completely through the end zone, it does not score a point.
9) If a team successfully knocks down all 3 of the opponent's pins, it wins the game; otherwise, the team with the most points at the end of the playing period would be the winner.

TEACHING SUGGESTIONS

1) After the first throw, balls are thrown back and forth at will. Players try to prevent balls from crossing their end zone, but may not go into the end zone to block or catch the ball. Players, otherwise, may move about freely within their own side of the playing area, but not enter opponent's territory. Players may run with the ball to the center line before throwing.
2) Teachers should encourage all students to throw the ball and not pass it to the best throwers. This way all students are getting ball throwing practice.

OUT BALL

1) Class forms one large circle and 2 balls are used (may be the same or different type balls) to pass around the circle from student to student.
2) Balls should be on opposite halves of the circle to begin with.
3) Whenever the instructor blows his or her whistle, the persons holding the ball in their hands receive an "O" (first letter in word "Out") against them, and then the game continues.
4) Once a person has received an O U T against them, they must step into the center of the circle. This person or persons must stay in the center until another player or players have received an O U T against them.
5) They would then change places and the person or persons going back to the circle would start clean without any letters against them.
6) Each person must handle the balls in turn.
7) Encourage students to turn to their left after passing a ball so that they are ready to catch the next ball when it is passed to them. With 2 balls the game moves fast and is rather suspenseful for the students.

5-AROUND

1) Divide the class in half with each group or team forming a circle.
2) The 2 circles will compete against each other, using whatever type of ball the teacher wishes to use.
3) One person in each circle will hold the ball for his or her circle over his/her head and upon the signal to start will pass the ball to the person on his/her right. When the ball has traveled around the circle once to the person who started it, everyone in that circle will yell "one!".
4) Each circle will continue to pass the ball around in the same direction and each time it reaches the head person the group will yell out the repetition, for example, "2", then 3, and so on, until the number called for has been reached, either 5-around or 10-around.
5) The first circle to successfully complete the number of cycles will be the winner.
6) Each person must handle the ball each time it travels around the circle, or the circle is disqualified.
7) They must pass the ball, not hand it to the person!

ZIGZAG DANISH ROUNDERS

1) One ball for each group. Approximately 6 students per group (3 facing 3).
2) Players in each group pass the ball back and forth in a zigzag pattern down the line and back within their own group.
3) On the whistle, the player with the ball holds the ball and the other players in his or her group line up behind him/her. As the players line up, the ball is handed overhead from player to player.
4) The last player in line runs up to the head of his/her line and calls "Danish Rounders".
5) The group finishing first, wins.
6) Each player must hand the ball, it cannot be thrown. If the ball is dropped, it is started again at the point it was dropped.

TEACHING SUGGESTIONS

Vary the types of passes in the 2 lines: underhand, overhand, bounce, bowling, etc.
Vary the passing down the single line: overhead, under, over and under, etc.

DODGEBALL GAME CHALLENGES

INS AND OUTS

1) Half of the players are "Ins" and half are "Outs".
2) Ins are inside the circle and Outs are outside the circle.
3) Outs standing with both feet outside of the circle, try to hit Ins with the ball.
4) Ball must land below waist of the person who is hit.
5) When an "In" is hit, he/she joins the "Outs" and tries to hit other "Ins".
6) Winner is the "In" who stays in the circle the longest.
7) Game is repeated with the players who were "Ins" becoming "Outs", and "Outs" becoming "Ins".
8) The game may end in a "play-off" between the 2 winners, if desired, and a champion decided. Use 2 balls, either rubber or volleyballs.

BOMBER

1) 2 players are the "Bombers" and stand opposite each other outside of the circle.
2) Bombers try to hit other players with a ball.
3) A fair hit must land below the waist and the ball must have been thrown from outside the circle.
4) When a player is hit, he or she joins the "Bombers" on the outside of the circle and helps to hit the remaining players.
5) 2 players who remain longest in the circle become "Bombers" for the next game.

CIRCLE EXCHANGE BALL

1) 2 lines of players facing each other with a circle midway between the lines.
2) Players in each line count off so there will be 2 ones, 2 twos, etc.
3) An "it" stands in the center circle with a volleyball in the left hand (or opposite throwing hand).
4) The leader calls out the player's numbers and designated players attempt to switch places in the lines while "it" attempts to hit one of them with a left-handed throw of the volleyball. (Players switching places must run and dodge through the circle.)
5) A hit player exchanges place with the thrower and the thrower takes his or her number.
6) If no player is hit, the ball is returned to the thrower and the leader calls a new number.

PRISONER'S DODGEBALL

1) Players (works best for students in Grades 3 to 8) are divided into 2 equal teams with each team positioning itself in one-half of a rectangular court containing a center line and 2 end zones or prisons.
2) Each team has one volleyball or rubber ball in its possession when the whistle is blown to start the play.
3) Players throw the balls back and forth at each other across the center line, trying to hit an opponent below the waist with the ball.
4) If the ball hits an opponent before hitting the ground, then the player hit becomes a prisoner and goes across the center line to the opponent's prison.
5) If the hands or arms are hit while below the waist level, this counts as being hit below the waist.
6) Prisoners can be freed by securing a ball while still in prison and hitting an opponent below the waist with the ball.

7) Prisoner gets a free walk back to his or her own territory and the opponent hit must go to prison.
8) A prisoner cannot leave prison (with both feet out) to secure a loose ball. Penalty for this is to forfeit a player to prison from the prisoner's team. However, teammates may try to free prisoners by throwing the ball into the prison. *Prisoner still has to hit an opponent before he or she can go free.*
9) Opponents cannot step into a prison area when attempting to block or intercept the ball being passed to prisoners. They can, however, run through the prison to retrieve the balls which leave the game area.
10) The object of the game is to secure all of the opponents in your team's prison area.
11) A ball which is thrown out of bounds can only be retrieved by players from the team in whose court side the ball went out. Players may not duck down on knees to avoid being hit.

TEACHING SUGGESTIONS

For rule #8 above, you may wish to try a modification in which *only* prisoners are allowed to chase after the balls which pass completely through the prison area. Under this rule there would naturally be no penalty for going out of the prison and court area.

BALL WALL GAME CHALLENGES

Among the most exciting games to be played on elementary school playgrounds, are those involving the use of a wall for hitting balls against. "Ball Wall" type games require a considerable amount of hand-eye coordination skills, and enable students to become involved in challenging game activities that may be easily modified down to the skill level of the participants. The following 4 games are among the most popular and basic "Ball Wall" games played by elementary school students. All 4 of the games presented require a wall and a rubber ball.

WALL BALL

SKILLS

1) Striking ball against wall (1 or 2 hands)
2) Positioning for proper return of ball

RULES

1) Two players stand facing the wall. All other players are lined up in the challenge or waiting line outside of the court area.
2) The player with the ball who starts the game, drops the ball and using one or two hands (open or closed) strikes the ball against the wall. (This player is called the "server".) NOTE: For older children at higher skill levels, the server should put the ball in play from behind the half court line.
3) The second player who is the receiver must return (strike) the ball against the wall before it bounces more than once on the ground. NOTE: Ball may hit the wall either above or below line painted across the wall.
4) The ball may be hit on the fly (before it bounces) or after one bounce. Players may use one or two hands.
5) The two players continue to alternate hitting the ball against the wall until one player fails to either: a) Hit the ball; b) Fails to reach the wall directly (no bounce); c) Has too many bounces (more than one) before returning the ball; d) Hits a ball against wall which lands outside the court area (liners are "out", the same

as in 4-Square); or e) Fails to move out of the way after hitting the ball, and interferes with opponents opportunity to hit the ball.

6) The player violating a rule is the loser of the game and goes to the end of the waiting or challenge line.
7) The new player (challenger) serves first and play continues.

CHINESE HANDBALL

SKILLS

1) Striking ball so that it bounces and then hits the wall
2) Positioning for proper return of ball

RULES

1) The same rules as listed for "Wall Ball" apply to Chinese Handball with the following exceptions:
   a) Server begins play by striking ball with open or closed hand(s) so that the ball *bounces one time* before hitting the wall. (Ball cannot be hit directly against the wall. It must bounce off the ground and hit the wall.)
   b) The receiver must strike the ball before it bounces twice, and return the ball so that it bounces one time and hits the wall.
2) Receiver may strike the ball after a direct rebound off the wall ("on the fly") as in "Wall Ball".
3) Play continues in this same manner with each player alternately hitting the ball until player commits a fault.
4) Winner stays on court and next player in waiting line (challenger) begins play by serving the ball.

THROW AND CATCH REBOUND BALL

SKILLS

1) Throwing ball against wall
2) Catching ball rebounding from wall
3) Positioning for catching the ball

SPECIAL NOTATION

This game is a modified version of "Wall Ball" and "Chinese Handball", and involves throwing and catching the ball. It is designed for younger children who have *not* yet mastered the skill of striking (hitting) the ball with control.

RULES

1) The same rules as listed for "Wall Ball" apply with the following exceptions:
   a) Server puts ball into play by throwing it against the wall using one or two hands. NOTE: Players start play from behind center court (or half court) line.
   b) Opponent (receiver) must catch the ball before it bounces more than once on the ground.
   c) Receiver has the option of catching the ball before it bounces ("on the fly") or after one bounce.
2) Play continues in this same manner with one player throwing the ball against the wall and one player catching the ball.
3) Winner stays on court and next player in waiting line (challenger) begins play by throwing (serving) ball from behind center court line.

ALTERNATE RULE

Depending on skill level, it is usually best to require that the ball must hit the wall above the "foul" line normally painted across the wall.

STRIDE-JUMP BALL

SKILLS

1) Throwing and catching ball
2) Stride-Jumping

FORMATION

Three players numbered in order line up behind the center court line.

RULES

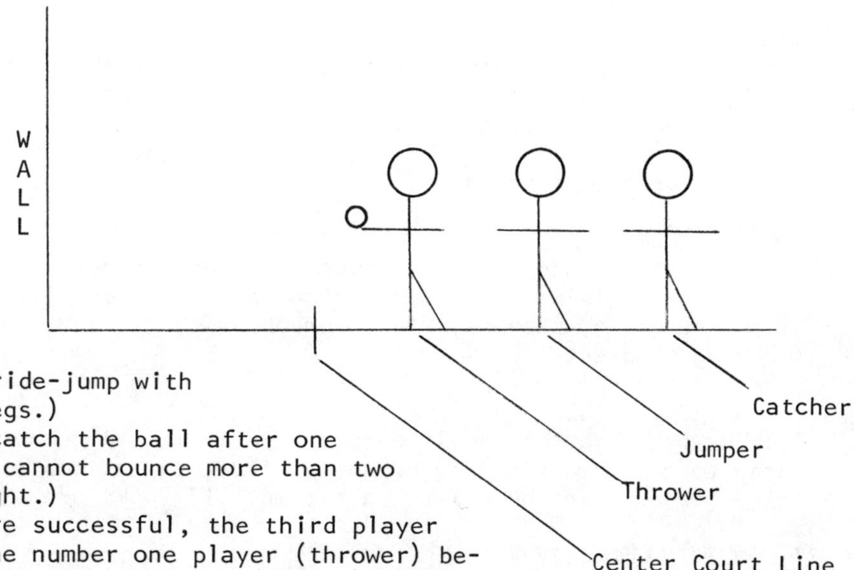

1) First player in line (see diagram at right) throws ball directly against the wall using an overhand throw. The ball must rebound once in front of the center court line.
2) The second player in order performs a stride-jump over the ball as it bounces. (Legs come apart on stride-jump with ball passing between legs.)
3) The third player must catch the ball after one or two bounces. (Ball cannot bounce more than two times before being caught.)
4) If all three players are successful, the third player becomes the thrower, the number one player (thrower) becomes the jumper, and the second player (jumper) becomes the receiver (or catcher).
5) If a player misses at his/her numbered position this player goes to the end of the waiting or challenger's line outside the court area. Example: Number two player fails to stride-jump the ball as it bounces, or number three player fails to catch the ball after one or two bounces.
6) A new player entering the game from the waiting line becomes the catcher or third position player. Players remaining in the game move accordingly.

PERCEPTION GAME CHALLENGES

VISUAL DISCRIMINATION

WHAT IS MISSING?

6 to 9 objects are arranged in a row on a table or chalkboard ledge, as students watch. Students then cover their eyes. Teacher removes one or 2 objects. A student is then asked what has been taken away.

WHAT IS THIS SHAPE?

Teacher "draws in the air" a large outline of some object in the room. Students are asked to look around and guess what was outlined. Sometimes hints as to the location of the objects are needed. Teacher may also draw in the air numbers or letters of the alphabet and call on students to identify the correct one.

FIND A SHAPE LIKE THIS

Teacher shows a cardboard circle form. A student is asked to touch everything in sight in the room that is the same shape (or give the student a definite number of objects to touch that are the same shape). Teacher then uses a square, rectangle, triangle, etc.

EACH IN ITS PLACE

Teacher or student arranges 3, 4, or 5 objects in a row, while the rest of the group covers their eyes. Students look at the objects for several seconds. Then one is called on to face the class (turning his or her back toward a row of objects), and name them in order, while other students watch. Order of the objects is then changed.

HIDE AWAY

Using a brown paper bag (or a large basket), teacher goes around the classroom, holding up objects, then placing them in a bag. One student is chosen to tell what is in the bag; another takes objects out. The rest of the class is involved, for the students are asked to give hints. This game will be enjoyed more if the teacher and the students bring a variety of things to put in the bag.

TOUCH 4 PEOPLE

Teacher goes around the room, touching 4 or 5 people. A student is asked to tell who was touched, giving the names in the correct order. If the student can't remember, hints are given, such as, "It's someone with red on". A variation of this game would be touching 4 objects.

GET SOMETHING BIGGER

Teacher places a very small object on a table. A number of students are called on, in turn, to get something bigger and place it on the table. It is fun to try to get something larger than the object each time. If rocks are available, it is especially fun.

GET SOMETHING SMALLER

This is the preceding game in reverse.

ONE FROM THE RING

Have the students sit in a circle (ring). Place balls (or other group of objects) of different colors in the center. The students hide their eyes while one student removes one of the balls. The object of the game is to tell which color ball has been removed. The student who is called upon, and knows the correct color, has the next turn. The difficulty of the game is, of course, determined by the number of balls placed in the center.

I SPY

The teacher describes an object without mentioning its name. The students look around the room until they locate the object which the teacher described. The first one to say, "I Spy", and who correctly identifies the object, has the next turn to describe something in the classroom.

AUDITORY DISCRIMINATION

WHO HAS THE CASTANET?

One student stands in front of the room with back turned to the group. Another student is given the castanet. All students keep hands behind their back and pretend to be shaking the castanet. The student who is the guesser turns and listens for the castanet. He or she then attempts to guess who has the castanet. You may wish to use a bell or other type of noise maker.

FINISHING RHYMES

Teacher repeats a rhyme. The 2nd and 3rd times, the students come in with the last words as the teacher stops. For example, "Hickery, Dickery, __________, the mouse ran up the _________". Start with familiar rhymes.

SECURING OBJECTS

Teacher asks: "Who would like to try to get 4 things that we mention?" The teacher then names, for example, a book, a ball, a top, and a piece of paper. A student goes and gets the 4 things. If there are the "makings" of a grocery store or toy store in the room, the game could be played "doing an errand at the store". Another variation would be to give the names of 4 people and have a student tap them in the order named.

MOVEMENT SEQUENCES

Teacher verbally gives movement directions to a student or class and they attempt to respond in the correct order. For example, the teacher can say: "Take 2 steps forward, turn around, then clap twice", and so on. This is excellent sequential memory training.

TAP THE RHYTHM

Teacher taps a rhythmic beat. One student, then the whole group, copies the beat. Rhythm sticks or pencils may be used, or students may clap the rhythm.

WHO IS IT?

A student in the class is described. Others try to guess who has been described.

NAME THE ANIMAL

Teacher places pictures of about 8 animals in plain view. The teacher describes one without naming it. A student is asked to come up and touch the animal described. Or, the teacher may read a rhyme about an animal without naming it. A good variation would be to let one student give the description. The game can be played with pictures of foods, homes, means of transportation, workers, tools, etc. Objects could be used instead of pictures.

LET'S ACT IT

Teacher tells a short story. Whenever there is action or facial expression indicated, the teacher says, "Let's all show what he or she did", or "Let's show how he or she looked".

WHAT SONG AM I TAPPING?

Teacher may mention the names of 3 familiar songs. She then taps the rhythm of several bars of one. Students try to guess which song it was.

WHAT DID I TAP?

Teacher goes around the room slowly, tapping each of 6 or 7 objects with a tom tom beater. (Objects would be of wood, metal, glass, cardboard.) Then the students cover their eyes. Teacher taps each one 3 times. A student is asked to identify one at a time by telling what type of object (cardboard, metal, etc.,) or by tapping the object. If the student is correct, he or she tries another.

HIGH, LOW, OR IN BETWEEN

Students cover their eyes. The teacher taps something up high. Students uncover their eyes and try to guess whether the object was high, low, or "in between". If just one student at a time is the guesser, the game goes better than having the whole class call out.

HIDE THE SPOOL

One student is sent from the room. When another has hidden a spool or other object, a doorkeeper invites the student to re-enter the room. The others indicate to the student where the object is by clapping their hands. If the student approaches the object, they clap softly, and if the student goes away from the object they begin clapping louder. If a student locates the object, he or she has the next turn to hide it.

LISTEN AND DO

At first, the students imitate the actions of the teacher. The teacher may put his or her hands on his or her head, shoulders, knees, behind the back, etc. Then the teacher says *one* thing, but does *another*. The students must follow the directions of the teacher's spoken words rather than imitate the actions. (This is similar to "Simon Says".)

EQUIPMENT DIAGRAMS

REBOUND NET

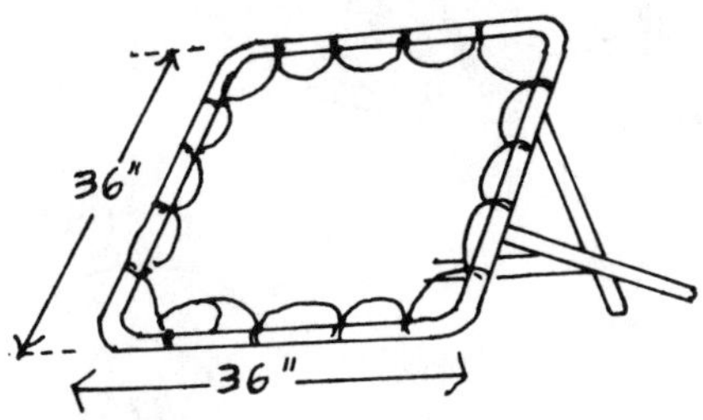

LAUNCHING BOARD

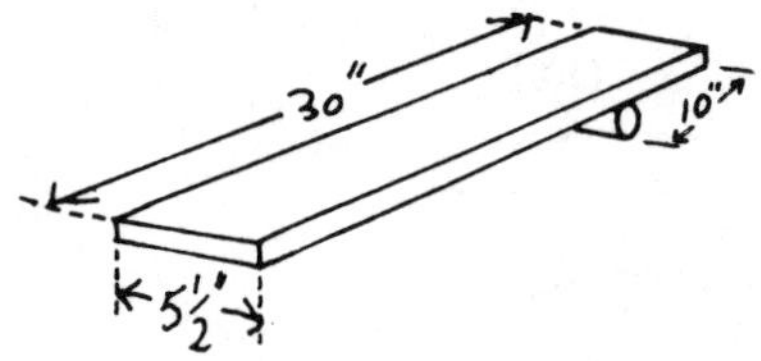

BICYCLE TIRE

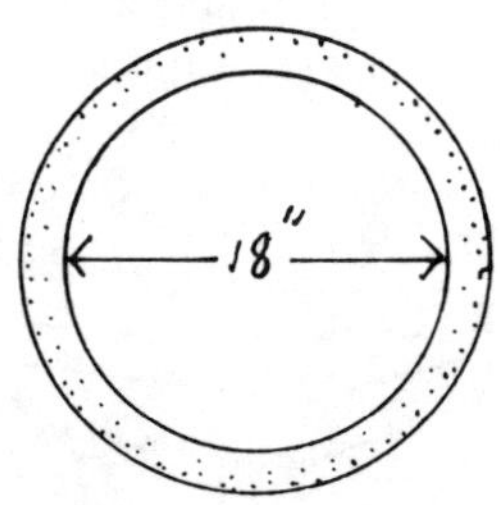

JUMP STANDARD

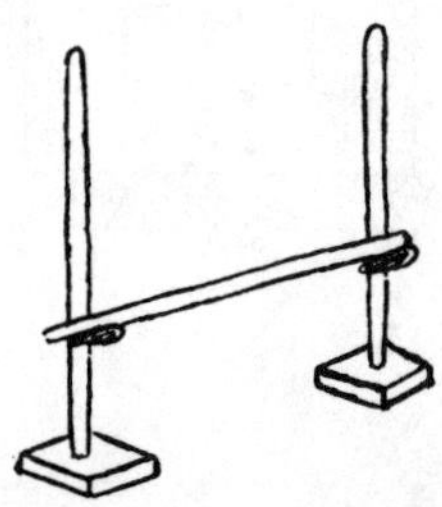

Jump Standard with cross bar placed over top of loops

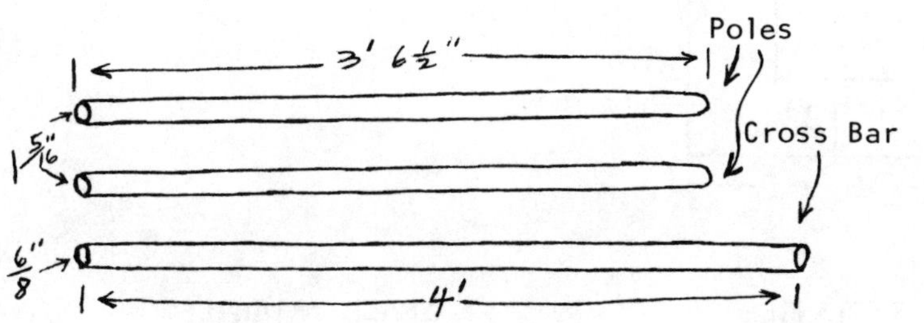

Pole & Cross Bar dimensions

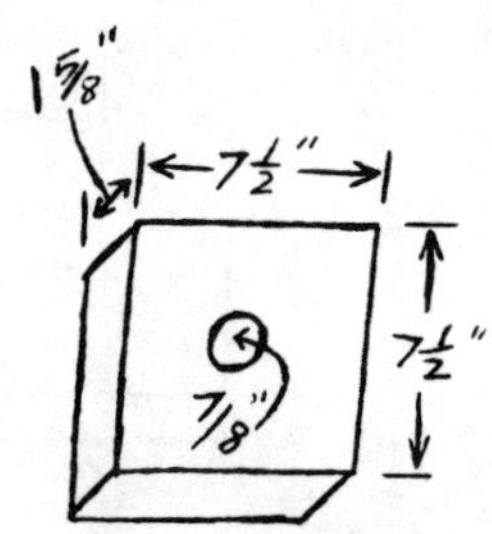

Base Support dimensions

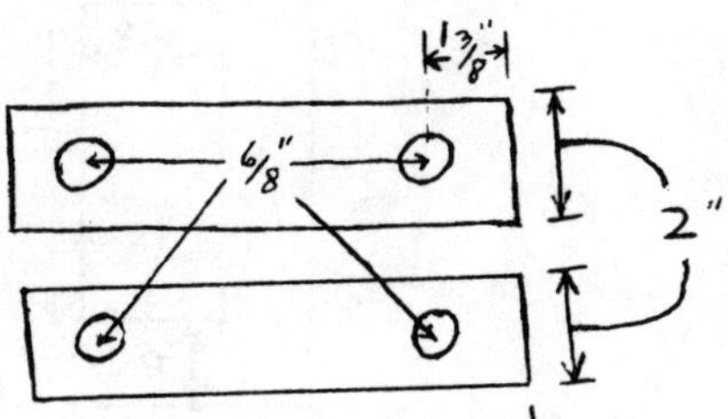

Loop dimensions

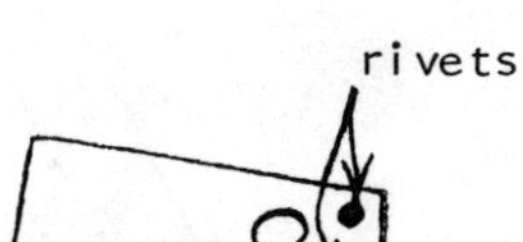

Loop folded in half and riveted together

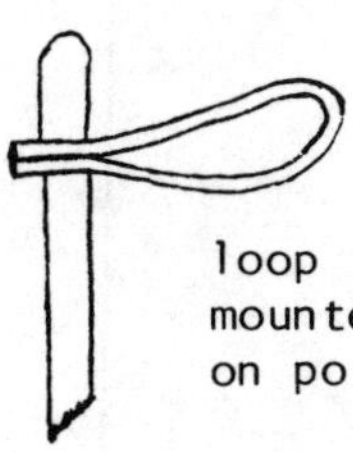

loop mounted on pole

GEOMETRIC SHAPES

Shapes are cut from 4 foot x 8 foot sheet of plywood 1/2 inch thick. Also, a 2nd proportionately larger triangle is cut from a separate piece of plywood. It's outside dimensions are 39 ½ inches each side, inside dimensions are 29 3/4 inches each side, and the width is the standard 3 inches.

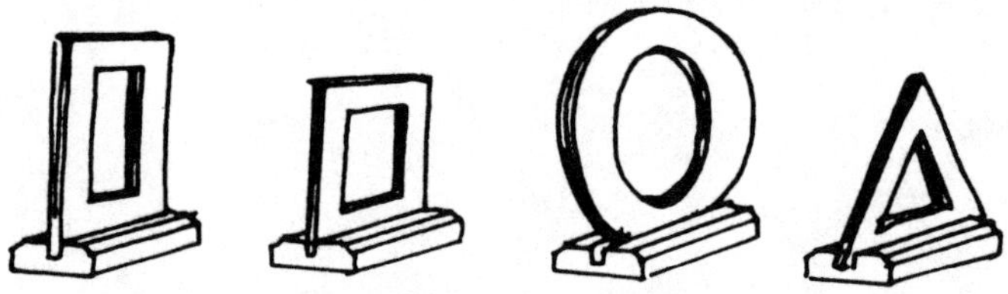

LARGE CIRCLE

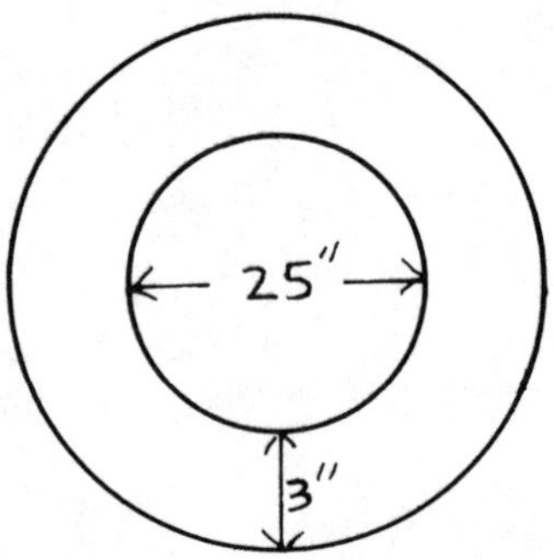

SMALL CIRCLE

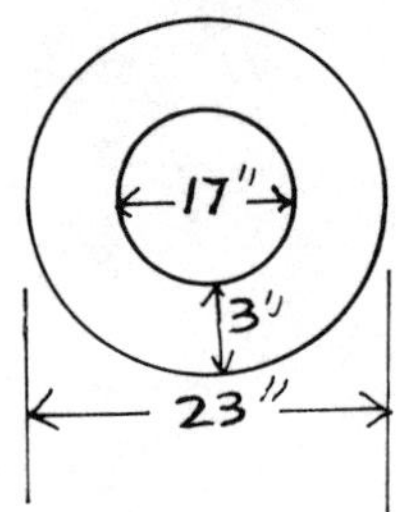

SUPPORT STAND FOR SHAPES

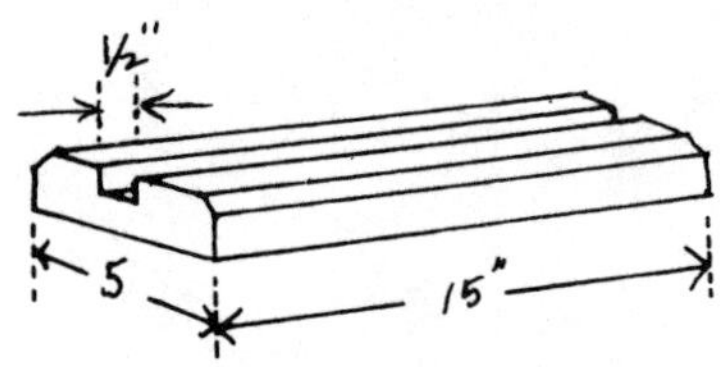

LARGE SQUARE

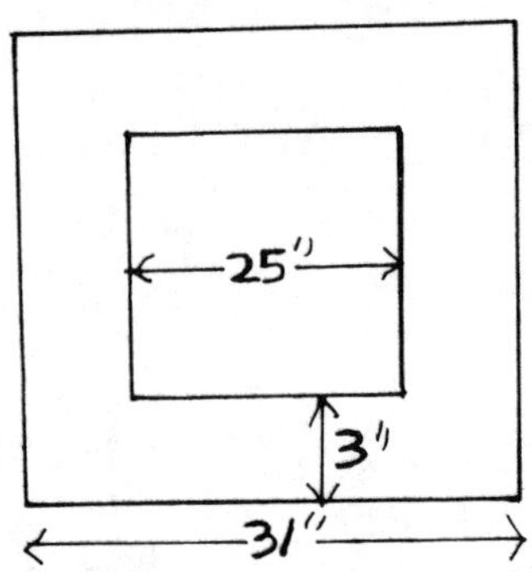

SMALL SQUARE

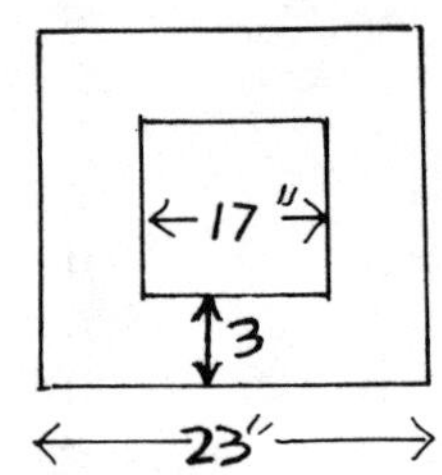

LARGE RECTANGLE

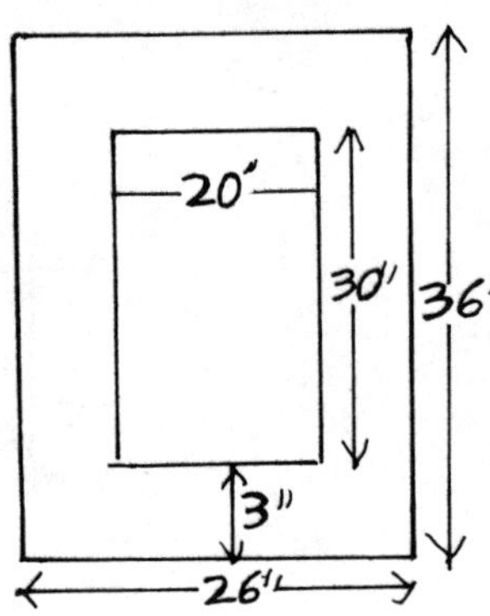

SMALL TRIANGLE

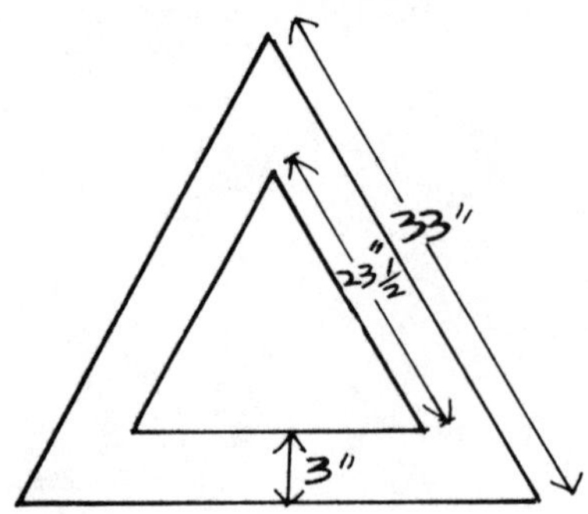

SMALL RECTANGLE

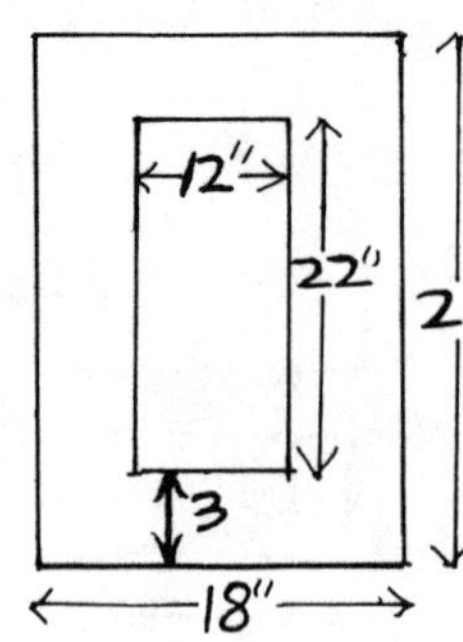

WALKING BOARD

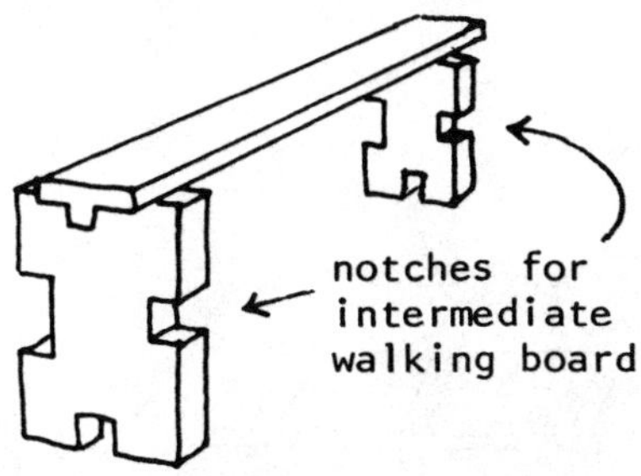

HIGH WALKING BOARD

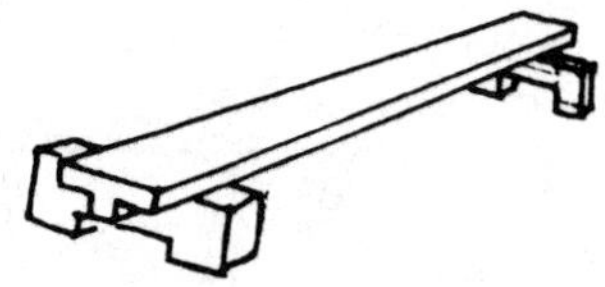

LOW WALKING BOARD

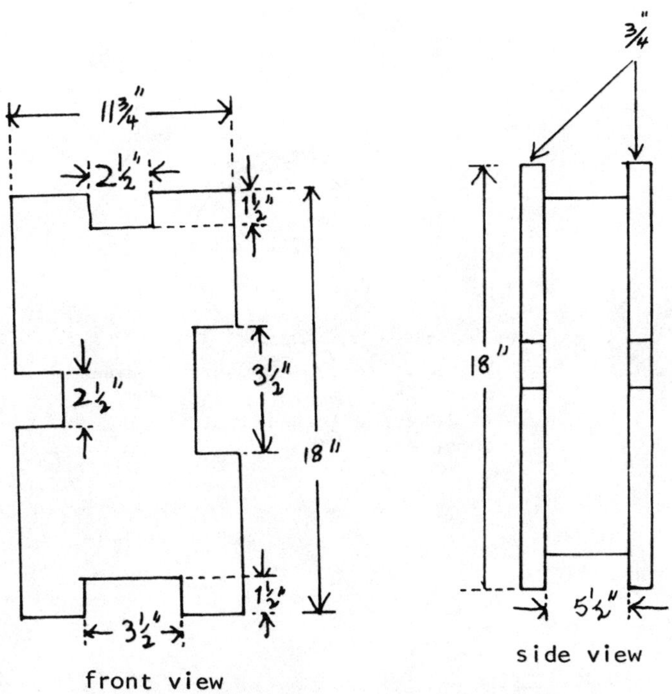

COMBINATION HIGH AND INTERMEDIATE WALKING BOARD SUPPORTS

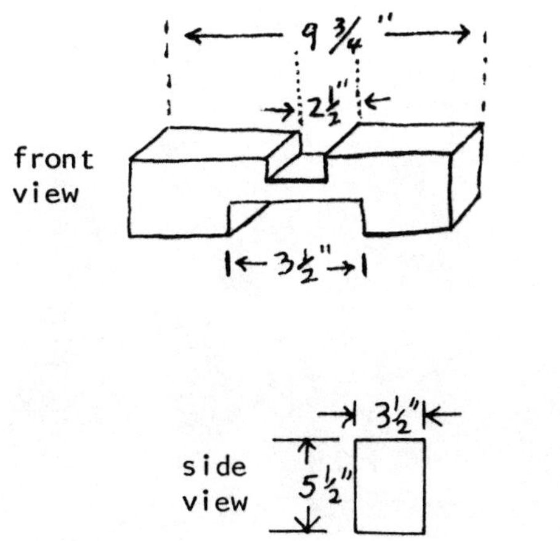

LOW WALKING BOARD SUPPORT

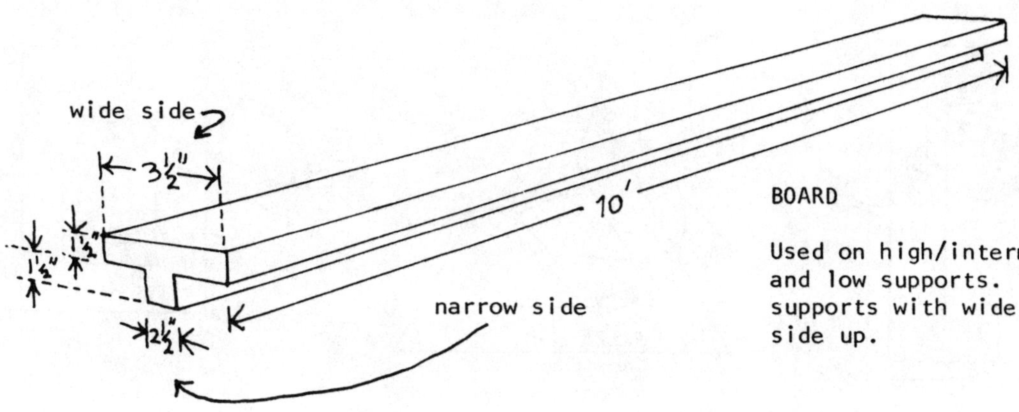

BOARD

Used on high/intermediate supports and low supports. Can be placed on supports with wide side up or narrow side up.

COORDINATION LADDER

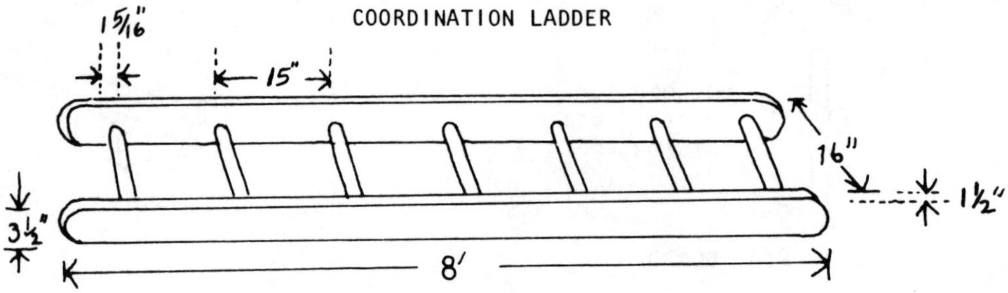

SCOOTER BOARD

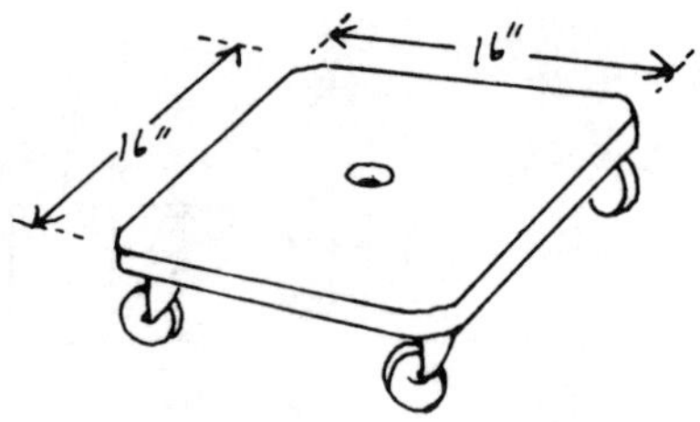

HOOP

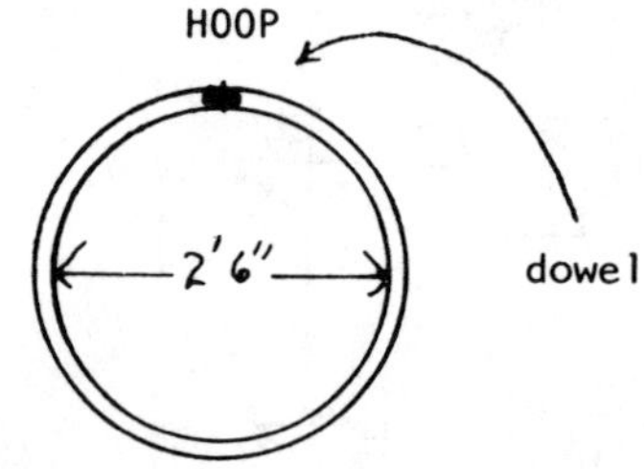

Use plastic pipe or tube 8' long with 3/4" diameter. Wood dowel is inserted to help hold hoop together.

CROSS BARS & TRAFFIC CONES

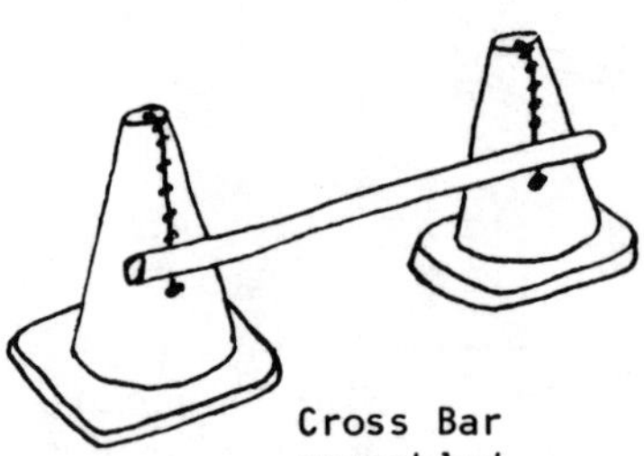

Cross Bar assembled

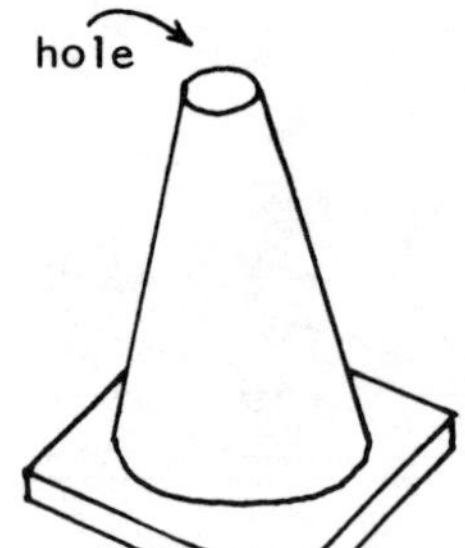

Traffic or Game Cone

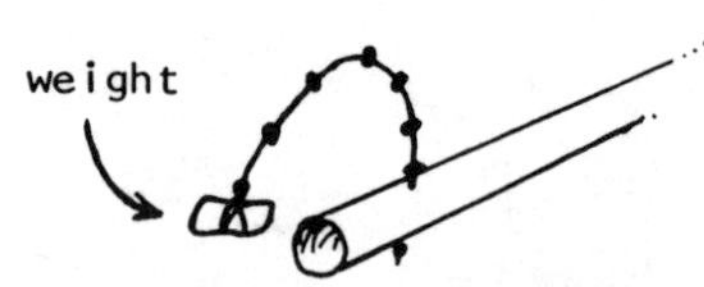

cross tube end with knotted cord and weight

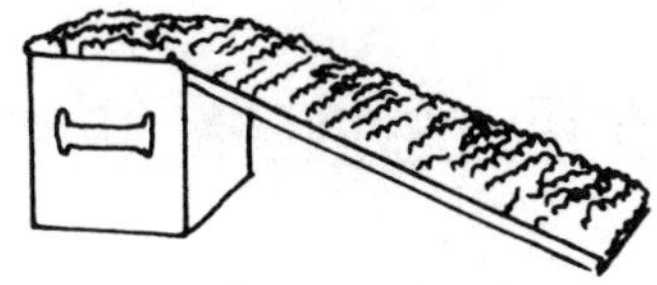

JUMP BOX

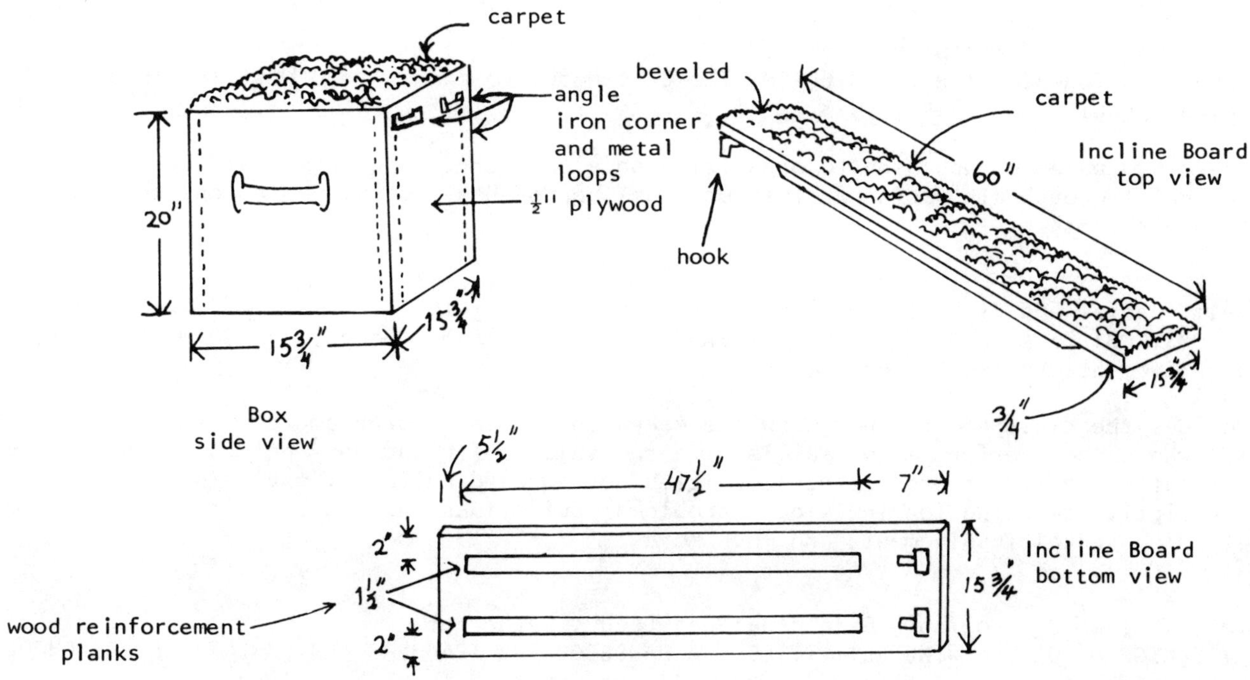

AUTO TIRE IN SUPPORT STAND

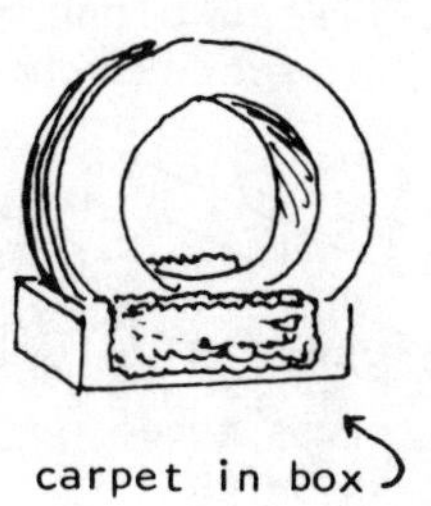

AUTO TIRE SUPPORT STAND

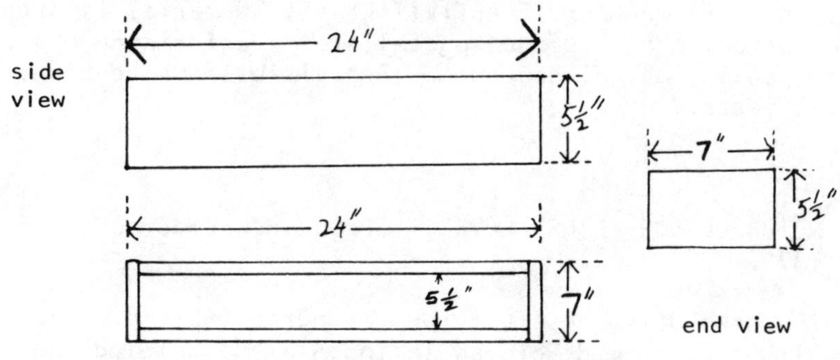

top view

RECOMMENDED MOTOR DEVELOPMENT RESOURCE BOOKS

Arnheim, Daniel and Pestolesi, Robert
DEVELOPING MOTOR BEHAVIOR IN CHILDREN, The C.V. Mosby Company, 11830 Westline Industrial Drive, St. Louis, Mo. 63141, 1973.

Presents a balanced approach to organizing an elementary school physical education program. Includes thorough discussion on instructional approaches, activity progression, and evaluating performance.

Arnheim, Daniel and Sinclair, William
THE CLUMSY CHILD: A PROGRAM OF MOTOR THERAPY, The C.V. Mosby Company, 11830 Westline Industrial Drive, St. Louis, Mo. 63141, 1975.

Provides the classroom teacher with the means to develop a program for working with children who cannot perform motor skills with the same proficiency as their classmates. Subject matter includes: organizing activities for awkward children; analysis of motor tests; prescriptive teaching for individual problems; guidelines for activity instruction; evaluation; parental involvement; and much more.

Braley, William T.; Konichi, Geraldine; and Leedy, Catherine
DAILY SENSORIMOTOR TRAINING ACTIVITIES. A HANDBOOK FOR TEACHERS AND PARENTS OF PRESCHOOL CHILDREN, Education Activities, P.O. Box 392, Freeport, L.I., N.Y. , 1968.

A resource book with activities designed to increase perceptual awareness and motor ability in young children. Activities are listed by perceptual abilities which need to be reinforced in the school and home environment. Good resource book for teachers and parents.

Capon, Jack J.
PERCEPTUAL MOTOR DEVELOPMENT, Pitman Learning, 6 Davis Drive, Belmont, CA 94002, 1975

A series of 5 books for preschool and elementary grades entitled: BASIC MOVEMENT ACTIVITIES, #1; BALL ROPE, HOOP ACTIVITIES # 2; BALANCE ACTIVITIES # 3; BEAN BAGS, RHYTHM STICK ACTIVITIES # 4; and TIRE, PARACHUTE ACTIVITIES #5. Material is organized for easy implementation by both classroom teachers and specialists. Performance objectives are listed along with tasks arranged in logical sequence. Activities have been child tested for success over a period of 8 years.

Capon, Jack J.
PERCEPTUAL-MOTOR LESSON PLANS, LEVEL-1, Front Row Experience, 540 Discovery Bay Blvd., Byron, Ca. 94514, 1975.

Includes 25 weeks of successfully proven perceptual-motor lesson plans sequenced according to difficulty. Program developed in the Alameda Unified School District, Alameda, Calif., and refined over a period of 8 years. Lessons are appropriate for preschool to first grade and special education classes. Contains perceptual-motor evaluation scale and equipment construction plans. Book is also published in a Station Card format to make it easier to implement the program.

Capon, Jack J.
PERCEPTUAL-MOTOR LESSON PLANS, LEVEL-2, Front Row Experience, 540 Discovery Bay Blvd., Byron, Ca. 94514, 1977.

Program designed for students who have successfully completed the basic Level-1 Program, but particularly appropriate for students in grades 2 and 3. Contains 25 weeks of successfully proven lesson plans. Each weekly plan contains 3 lesson phases: 1) Perceptual-motor lessons with 4 learning stations; 2) Movement exploration lessons; and 3) Game lessons. Contains evaluation scale and equipment construction plans. Book is also published in a Station Card format to make it easier to implement the program.

Cratty, Bryant
REMEDIAL MOTOR ACTIVITY FOR CHILDREN, Lea and Febiger Co., Washington Square, Philadelphia, Pa. 19106, 1975.

This text focuses upon the assessment and remediation of movement behavior problems. It is intended to provide a theoretical base, suggestions for evaluation, and guidelines and principles which undergrid remedial techniques and practices.

Cratty, Bryant J.
DEVELOPMENTAL SEQUENCES OF PERCEPTUAL-MOTOR TASKS, Education Activities, P.O. Box 392, Freeport, L.I., N.Y.

Directed towards neurologically handicapped and mentally retarded children, but material presented has great implications for all children. Appropriate movement activities are presented in sequence and listed under specific perceptual-motor characteristics.

Dauer, Victor P. and Pangrazi, Robert
DYNAMIC PHYSICAL EDUCATION FOR ELEMENTARY SCHOOL CHILDREN, Minneapolis: Burgess Publishing Company, 1968.

A comprehensive text and resource book for planning and conducting a broad physical education program with discussion on movement education and perceptual-motor training. Excellent publication!

Evans, Jack
STEGEL MOVEMENT ACTIVITIES, Front Row Experience, 540 Discovery Bay Blvd., Byron, Calif. 94514, 1978

Focus is on the various approaches to using the Stegel (also called the Lind Climber) in movement programs. Complete lesson plans are presented in sequence and include use of balance beams, parallel bars, climbing, jumping, vaulting, and general exploration. Detailed drawings are provided with each lesson in this fully illustrated book.

Flinchum, Betty
MOTOR DEVELOPMENT IN EARLY CHILDHOOD: A GUIDE FOR MOVEMENT EDUCATION - AGES 2-6, C.V. Mosby Co., 11830 Westline Industrial Dr., St Louis, Mo. 63141, 1975

Movement plays a vital role in a child's development. This book provides the "what", "how", and "why" instruction of perceptual-motor skills for preschool children. It offers a knowledge base for observation and analysis of children's movement through basic taxonomy of fine and gross motor skills; and a pictorial analysis of selected skills.

Frostig, Marianne
MOVE-GROW-LEARN, Follett Educational Corporation, P.O. Box 5705, Chicago, Illinois 60680, 1969

Contains teacher's manual along with 181 exercise cards for teaching movement skills to preschool, kindergarten, and primary grade children. The program is designed to enhance the total development of young children. Activities are very basic, easy to interpret, and practical for implementation.

Furth, Hans and Wachs, Harry
THINKING GOES TO SCHOOL, Oxford University Press, Inc., 200 Madison Ave, N.Y., N.Y. 10016

This unique book includes a review of Piaget's theories along with extensive coverage of thinking games and activities which will help children to develop sensory and perceptual-motor processes. General areas covered include "General Movement Thinking", "Visual Thinking", "Auditory Thinking", "Hand Thinking", etc.

Gallahue, David; Werner, Peter; and Luedke, George
A CONCEPTUAL APPROACH TO MOVING AND LEARNING, John Wiley and Sons, Inc., N.Y. 1975

Focuses on fundamental and general movement concepts that need to be developed by preschool and elementary age children. A structural model showing 6 stages of motor development is presented and discussed. The book examines 3 categories of movement: Locomotion, Manipulation, and Stability.

Gilbert, Anne
TEACHING THE THREE R'S THROUGH MOVEMENT EXPERIENCES, Burgess Publishing Co., 7108 Ohms Lane, Minneapolis, Mn 55435, 1977.

Describes how movement experiences can be used in traditional academic subjects to introduce, reinforce, and review basic learning concepts. An excellent book on activities for integration of movement into the total school curriculum.

Hackett, Layne C. and Jenson, Robert G.
A GUIDE TO MOVEMENT EXPLORATION, Peek Publications, Box 11065, Palo Alto, Ca. 94306, 1966.

A discussion of the goals and methods of implementing movement exploration. Describes procedures for using implements such as balls, hoops, ropes, tires, etc. Includes suggested daily, weekly, and yearly lesson plans for grades K-6.

Kirchner, Glenn
PHYSICAL EDUCATION FOR ELEMENTARY SCHOOL CHILDREN, William C. Brown Co., Dubuque, Iowa, 1969.

An excellent book showing the many ways of incorporating movement experiences for children into the physical education program. A good analysis of various movement skills and activities in the elementary program is provided with many illustrations.

Lerch-Becker-Ward-Nelson
PERCEPTUAL-MOTOR LEARNING - THEORY AND PRACTICE, Peek Publications, Box 11065, Palo Alto, Ca. 94306, 1974.

Excellent section on theory behind the perceptual-motor programs along with implications of research studies. A review of various screening instruments is included as well as resource lists of books, records, and films. Activities are presented in a very practical way and include diagrams.

McCullock, Lovell
A HANDBOOK FOR DEVELOPING PERCEPTUAL-MOTOR AND SENSORY SKILLS THROUGH BODY MOVEMENT, Austin Writers Group, P.O. Box 12642 Capitol Stations, Austin, Texas 78711, 1973.

A comprehensive resource book covering perceptual-motor skills activities, gross-motor experiences, and sensory-motor integration skills. Sample lesson plans and equipment diagrams are included. Very extensive and well organized.

O'Quinn, Garland
GYMNASTICS FOR ELEMENTARY SCHOOL CHILDREN, University Stores, Inc., P.O. Box 1441, Austin, Texas 78767, 1973.

Lists step-by-step progression for using a variety of low cost gymnastics equipment items. Explanations are brief and easy to follow along with excellent pictures. Activities are carefully sequenced to provide positive results. Excellent publication!

Wickstrom, Ralph
FUNDAMENTAL MOTOR PATTERNS, (2nd Edition), Lea and Febiger, Washington Square, Phildelphia, PA 19106, 1977

A revised and updated edition on fundamental motor patterns. Stages and trends in motor development are clearly interpreted. The focus is on 7 basic movement skills: Walking, Running, Jumping, Throwing, Catching, Kicking, and Striking. An outstanding publication!

FOUNDATIONS AND PRACTICES IN PERCEPTUAL-MOTOR LEARNING - A QUEST FOR UNDERSTANDING, American Association For Health, Physical Education, Recreation, And Dance, 1201 16th St. N.W., Washington, D.C., 1971.

The material for this well organized and informative publication was obtained from speeches, discussions, and papers presented at the first national conference on Perceptual-Motor Development held in Cincinnati, Ohio, October, 1970. This valuable resource book also contains up-to-date information on Assessment Instruments, Innovative Programs, Research, and Films.

IMPROVING MOTOR-PERCEPTUAL SKILLS, Division of Continuing Education, Oregon State System of Higher Education, Waldo Hall 100, Corvallis, Oregon 97331, 1970.

IMPROVING MOTOR-PERCEPTUAL SKILLS, Division of Continuing Education, Oregon State System of Higher Education, Waldo Hall 100, Corvallis, Oregon 97331, 1970.

This step-by-step teacher's guide provides directions for conducting 34 classroom activities to increase children's physical and perceptual skills. The activities are grouped into 4 categories: general coordination, balance, body image, and eye-hand coordination. An extremely well organized, easy to use publication!